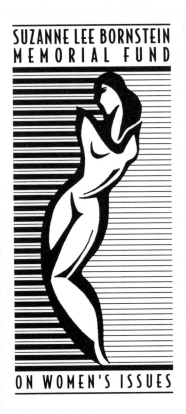

SUZANNE LEE BORNSTEIN
MEMORIAL FUND

ON WOMEN'S ISSUES

SCIENCE ON TRIAL

Science on Trial

THE CLASH OF MEDICAL EVIDENCE AND THE LAW IN THE BREAST IMPLANT CASE

Marcia Angell, M.D.

W. W. NORTON & COMPANY

LONDON

NEW YORK

For information about permission to reproduce selections from this book,
write to Permissions, W. W. Norton & Company, Inc.,
500 Fifth Avenue, New York, NY 10110.

The text of this book is composed in ITC New Baskerville with the display
set in Spartan Heavy Classified & ITC New Baskerville
Composition and manufacturing by the Haddon Craftsmen, Inc.
Book design by Beth Tondreau Design

LIBRARY OF CONGRESS CATALOGING-IN-PUBLICATION DATA
Angell, Marcia.
Science on trial : the clash of medical evidence and the law in
the breast implant case / Marcia Angell.
p. cm.
Includes bibliographical references and index.
ISBN 0-393-03973-0
1. Products liability—Breast implants—United States. 2. Breast implants—Law
and legislation—United States. 3. Breast implants—Complications.
I. Title.
KF1297.B74A96   1996
346.7303'8—dc20
[347.30638]   95-50081
CIP

W. W. Norton & Company, Inc., 500 Fifth Avenue, New York, N.Y. 10110
http://web.wwnorton.com

W. W. Norton & Company Ltd., 10 Coptic Street, London WC1A 1PU

1 2 3 4 5 6 7 8 9 0

To Lara and Elizabeth,
once again with love

CONTENTS

PREFACE

A few years ago I would have been surprised to be told I would one day write a book about breast implants. I had no particular interest in the subject, and it would have seemed unlikely that I would develop one. To be sure, as a physician I was aware that cosmetic surgery was a part of health care. But I considered it a relatively minor part, dwarfed by the many more crucial matters facing doctors and patients—life-threatening disease, unremitting pain, profound disability. Nor would my responsibilities as executive editor of the *New England Journal of Medicine* have been likely to involve me in the study of breast implants. My job is to help evaluate the many reports of medical research submitted to the *Journal*, of which only about 10 percent are selected for publication. Reports of breast implant research were rarely among the submissions and, until recently, never among the papers selected for publication. Not very much research was being done on the subject, and what there was wasn't very good. So how did the idea for this book come to be?

The short answer is that I was drawn to the issue by two manuscripts submitted to the *Journal*, one in 1992 and the second in 1994. In 1992 David Kessler, the commissioner of the FDA, banned silicone-gel-filled breast implants from the market because they had not been proven safe. The ban caused widespread alarm among the 1 million to 2 million women who already had implants. It also led to a torrent of lawsuits against the manufacturers of breast implants. Shortly after Kessler announced the ban, he submitted a manuscript to the *New England Journal of Medicine* explaining his reasons. In reviewing the manuscript I began to realize that the matter was more complicated than I had suspected. Kessler's decision involved not just science, but public opinion, politics, and the law. I thought the consequences of the FDA's decision would be far more wide-ranging than Kessler seemed to believe, and I wrote an editorial to that effect to accompany his article. That was my first exposure to the subject.

Two years later, in 1994, Dr. Sherine Gabriel of the Mayo Clinic submitted to the *New England Journal of Medicine* her report of the first epidemiologic study of whether breast implants increase the risk of certain diseases and symptoms. By this time, thousands of lawsuits had been filed alleging that they did. Some women received huge damages from sympathetic juries (the record was $25 million). For every jury verdict, many more cases were settled for the plaintiff out of court. The situation became unsustainable for the breast implant manufacturers, and so they agreed to set aside $4.25 billion to meet the claims of all women with breast implants once and for all—the biggest class-action settlement in history. Yet the Mayo Clinic study, published shortly after the class-action settlement was announced, did not show a link between breast implants and disease. I was struck by the discrepancy between the legal findings and the scientific evidence. Why were the courts so sure, when the scientists were not at all certain? I suggested some possible answers to this question in another editorial, which accompanied the Mayo Clinic study. That was my second foray into the subject, and by this time I was hooked.

But the most important reason I decided to write about

the breast implant controversy is because it illuminates important themes in American life. It richly illustrates the interplay of regulation, litigation, commercial interests, media coverage, and consumer pressure in the public confrontation of a major health issue. In the decade leading up to the FDA ban, the safety of implants was debated in the courts, in medical journals, and in the popular media. The debate occurred against a political backdrop of controversy about the relative excesses of big business and government regulation. Were large corporations like Dow Corning, the leading manufacturer of breast implants, knowingly foisting off dangerous products on the public or were they responsibly meeting consumer demands? Should the FDA have moved more promptly to pull implants off the market or should women have been allowed to make their own choices? After the ban, the focus shifted to the courts, where matters of scientific fact were decided not by scientists, but by lawyers, juries, and judges. On what basis did they reach their conclusions? And what effect did public opinion have on the outcome? The media covered the controversy fully, if not always accurately, and the public took a lively interest in the matter. Did public opinion drive the FDA's actions and the courts' conclusions? And how was the unfolding of the breast implant story affected by greed and the expectation of personal profit? Vast amounts of money, not just the $4.25 billion in the original class-action settlement, are still at stake in the thousands of individual lawsuits that have been filed and will be filed.

What fascinated me most about the contradictory opinions and accusations, the frenetic legal activity, and the huge sums of money at stake was the question of evidence. As I investigated the subject, I realized that the breast implant controversy is simply one example of the difficulty we Americans have in dealing with scientific evidence, particularly on matters of health. We depend greatly on science and its technological fruits, we like to talk about what research shows and what it doesn't, we think we understand risks, but when it comes to the recurrent medical scares that sweep across the land like locusts, all our sophistication goes out the window. Just give us the conclusion, tell us whom to blame, and don't bother with the evidence.

In this book, I will use the breast implant story to illustrate the broader themes that concern me. How do scientists reach conclusions about questions of health risks, such as whether breast implants increase the chance of developing a disease? How does the legal system reach its conclusions about the same question? Do the differences in methods account for the vast differences in outcome? What are the essential distinctions in the way science, the law, and the public regard evidence, and what are the consequences for our society?

I will begin with a brief review of the breast implant controversy to provide the narrative. To set the context further, I will describe in some detail the implants themselves, as well as the history of breast augmentation and the more recent use of implants for reconstruction after cancer surgery. In the remaining chapters, I will widen the focus to the themes illustrated by the breast implant story: the role of regulation and litigation in American life, the nature of scientific evidence, the way in which legal evidence is different, the distorting effect of greed and corruption on the usual process for deciding medical matters, the public's all-or-nothing response to health news, and the ripple effects of a paroxysm like the breast implant controversy.

Finally, a brief personal note to give the reader some idea of the point of view I bring to this subject. I consider myself a feminist, by which I mean that I believe that women should have political, economic, and social rights equal to those of men. As such, I am alert to discriminatory practices against women, which some feminists believe lie at the heart of the breast implant controversy. I am also a liberal Democrat. I believe that an unbridled free market leads to abuses and injustices and that government and the law need to play an active role in preventing them. Because of this view, I am quick to see the iniquities of large corporations. I disclose my political philosophy here, because it did not serve me well in examining the breast implant controversy. The facts were simply not as I expected they would be. But my most fundamental belief is that one should follow the evidence wherever it leads. From time to time, it is important to look up and see where you have been led and who is there with you, but you should not turn back. That is what this book is all about.

MARCIA ANGELL

ACKNOWLEDGMENTS

I could not have written this book without Rachel Hart, my extraordinary research assistant. Even before I put the first word on paper, she had assembled a voluminous file of information on the breast implant controversy, which she continually supplemented and revised as events unfolded. As my eyes and ears, and often my brain, she stayed in touch with many of the principals in the saga, and tried to make certain that no aspect of the controversy escaped us and that all our facts were accurate. She also performed the onerous task of writing endnotes for the chapters, so that interested readers might follow the same trail we did. And finally, she went over the book many times, offering insightful comments. It was my good fortune that she cared as much as I did.

I am also extremely grateful to Dr. Jerome Kassirer, the editor-in-chief of the *New England Journal of Medicine*, for his unwavering support, encouragement, and friendship as I struggled to fit together the schedules of writing the book and editing the *Journal*. The Massachusetts Medical Society, owners of the *New England Journal of Medicine*, also backed me fully. The executive vice-president, Dr. Harry Greene, enthusiastically agreed to free me for four months to write, and he was always available to offer advice and encouragement—but only if I asked for it. The legal staff of the *Journal*, especially Paul Auffermann, willingly provided whatever counsel I asked for during the preparation of the book. No one could work for more supportive people.

The following people were kind enough to read sections of the book and offer comments or expert advice: Bert Black, John Getter, Shirley Hufstedler, Sheridan Kassirer, Martha Minow, David Pate, Noel Rose, and Walter Willett. I am very grateful to them. In addition, I received helpful information or advice from Sherine Gabriel, Charles Hennekens, Deborah Hensler, Matthew Liang, Frank Speizer, and Richard Wilson. Hilary Hinzmann of W. W. Norton was a thoughtful and attentive editor. I am also indebted to my talented friend Darcy Tromanhauser, of Henry Holt, who provided a crash course in book publishing and led me to my capable agent, Alice Martell.

Bud Relman, my ultimate editor and partner in all things, carefully read every word in the book and changed many of them. His attention to the story I was telling and the way I told it was invaluable. More important, his enthusiasm for the project, along with the encouragement of my daughters, Lara and Elizabeth Goitein, kept me at it. They were a great home team.

MARCIA ANGELL

SCIENCE ON TRIAL

1

THE
BREAST IMPLANT
STORY:
ONCE OVER
LIGHTLY

B y the time FDA commissioner David Kessler decided in 1992 to ban silicone-gel-filled breast implants, an estimated 1 million to 2 million American women already had them.[1] (The precise number is unknown.) According to Kessler, the manufacturers had not fulfilled their responsibility to demonstrate the safety of the implants, and he therefore had no choice but to take them off the market. Thus ended 30 years of the easy availability of breast implants (for those who could afford the surgery). Most women with implants had simply wanted to enlarge their breasts, but about 20 percent had obtained them for reconstruction after mastectomy for breast cancer.[2] A 1990 survey commissioned by the American Society of Plastic and Reconstructive Surgeons found that over 90 percent of women with breast implants were well pleased with the results. Nevertheless, many people were jubilant about the FDA ban—including advocates of tough government regulation, women who believed breast implants had caused them to become ill, and feminists who thought it was about time someone put a stop to women being pressured to conform to male fantasies. What follows is the story of the breast implant controversy. It is an astonishing story, with implications far beyond the question of whether or not silicone-gel-filled breast implants are safe.

As executive editor of the *New England Journal of Medicine* and as a woman, I was aware that breast implants were controversial on many counts, but I had not given the matter much thought until Dr. Kessler submitted an article to the *Journal* explaining his reasons for banning the devices. The article was important and we were happy to publish it.[3] Still, I was troubled by the likely consequences of Kessler's action, as well as by some of his arguments. He seemed disdainful of women who wanted breast implants for purely cosmetic reasons, and his decision, though welcomed by many women, struck me as a little patronizing. More important, how would the sudden ban strike the million or so women who already had implants? Would they accept Kessler's legalistic argument that he was simply responding to the lack of evidence adduced by the manufacturers? I thought not. Far more likely, they would see the FDA ban as proof that the implants were extremely dangerous.

And that is exactly what happened. Despite Kessler's weak assurances that removal of the implants was unnecessary, women rushed to have them taken out, sometimes by the same plastic surgeons who had implanted them in the first place. One woman who could not afford the fee attempted to remove her own implants with a razor blade; she survived the ordeal, and was pictured in newspapers looking greatly relieved after a surgeon had finished the job.[4] Most notably, the small trickle of high-stakes court cases that began in the early 1980s swelled to a torrent.[5] Compassionate juries awarded multimillion-dollar damages to women with a variety of complaints that they and their lawyers attributed to breast implants.[6] If Kessler thought the ban was the end of the matter, he was wrong.

What *did* we know about the safety of breast implants? Kessler was right about this: at the time the FDA made its decision to ban them, we knew next to nothing. Incredibly, there had been no systematic studies of the effects of breast implants. We knew, of course, that there could be complications from the surgery itself (as with any surgery), including infections and hemorrhage. We also knew that in many women the tissue around the implants scarred excessively, distorting and hardening the breasts, and that these contractures could be uncomfortable. And finally, we knew that in a significant percentage of women (the best estimates are around 5 percent) an implant ruptured, releasing silicone gel into the surrounding tissues and flattening the breast.[7] But these local complications, unpleasant as they were, were not the basis for most of the alarm about breast implants, nor were they the focus of the multimillion-dollar lawsuits.

Instead, a growing number of Americans had come to believe that breast implants could cause devastating effects on the rest of the body. In particular, silicone-gel-filled implants were said to be responsible for a constellation of disorders known as connective tissue diseases. These diseases—which include systemic lupus erythematosus (SLE), rheumatoid arthritis, scleroderma, and polymyalgia, among others—are thought to involve a disturbance in the immune system that turns the body's protective defenses against itself. The result is an autoimmune disease—that is, a prolonged civil war within the body that can produce profound weakness and fatigue, along with variable damage to the joints, skin, and internal organs.

It was theorized that silicone, leaking slowly from the implants, provokes an immune reaction that then somehow turns into an autoimmune process. This theory, not the local complications, was the basis for most of the alarm and the largest lawsuits. Earlier worries that implants could cause cancer were largely eclipsed by the concern about connective tissue disease, in part because scientific studies were showing the cancer scare to be unfounded.[8] It is harder to study connective tissue disease than cancer, because it is more difficult to pin down or rule out the diagnosis.

Eventually, the breast implant manufacturers, losing one product liability case after another, agreed to the largest class-action settlement in the annals of American law.[9] Class actions are lawsuits in which the claims of many people are decided in a single court proceeding brought by representative plaintiffs. Through a class-action settlement, defendants can limit their losses by paying a set amount to be distributed among all those with a claim. In April 1994 the major manufacturers agreed to pay $4.25 billion to women with breast implants, a billion of which was explicitly set aside for the lawyers involved. Although nearly any woman with implants would be entitled to something under the terms of the settlement, women were permitted to opt out if they thought they could do better in court on their own. By June 1, 1995, 440,000 women had registered to participate in the class-action settlement (as many as a third of all women with breast implants in this country), but, with vigorous encouragement from plaintiffs' attorneys, about 15,000 (half Americans, half foreigners) had opted out to seek higher damages individually.

The implant manufacturers could have warned of a link between breast implants and connective tissue disease in the informational pamphlet they are required to put in each package of implants. If they had done so, they would have had less trouble. In addition to dissuading many women from considering implants, such a warning would have disarmed those who got implants anyway, since they could no longer have claimed that the manufacturers had misled them. A product liability suit is less likely to be successful if the buyer (in this case, the plastic surgeon, who is expected to inform the patient) has been warned. But the manufacturers steadfastly maintained that the implants were safe, despite the lack of scientific evidence in either direction. To be sure, there were many individual stories of connective tissue disease developing after the placement of breast implants, but these reports alone ("anecdotes," in scientific jargon) do not constitute evidence that the implants caused the disease. They could well have represented pure coincidence. Since connective tissue disease can develop in women with or without implants, the only way to demonstrate that implants actually cause the disease is to show that the risk is significantly higher in women *with* breast implants than it is in those *without* implants. To do so requires epidemiologic studies—scientific surveys of the incidence of disease in samples of different groups. But it was not until a few months after the class-action settlement was announced that the first such study of breast implants and connective tissue disease was published.[10]

How could the law have been so far out in front of the evidence that huge amounts of money were changing hands and $4.25 billion more was promised? And whose hands were they? Many of those who welcomed the FDA ban believed that the law was *not* in front of the evidence, but that the evidence had been largely suppressed by rapacious implant manufacturers interested only in their profits and by the plastic surgeons who made a very good living implanting the devices.

However, not even this conspiratorial theory does justice to the real complexity of the story. As suspected, the story is full of greed, but this greed is hardly limited to implant manufacturers and plastic surgeons. Plaintiffs' attorneys, doctors, researchers, and even implant recipients themselves are exploiting the lucrative opportunities. Four billion dollars is a lot of money, and there is even more to be had.

The breast implant story shows us some of the worst in human nature; it also reveals the weaknesses of a number of important U.S. institutions, including the media, parts of the legal and medical professions, and the courts. It raises the question of how we know what we think we know about the causes of disease, and, in so doing, it calls into question the systems we have devised for finding out. How *does* the public decide whether silicone breast implants or any other product is harmful? How do researchers and doctors decide, as compared with judges and juries? These issues can be considered within six broad themes that pervade and shape American society. All of the themes are clearly sounded in the breast implant controversy.

The first concerns the place of regulation in American life. The FDA, as perhaps the most visible of the governmental regulatory bodies, faced a virtually impossible dilemma in deciding whether or not to ban breast implants. Whatever its decision, the FDA would be strongly criticized. If implants were left on the market, the FDA would be seen as caving in to the manufacturers. If they were banned, at least a million women might wrongly conclude that they were at risk for serious disease. The letter of the law requires that manufacturers of devices demonstrate their safety before they market them. But breast implants had been on the market for a dozen years or so before that law was passed and another dozen afterward before the FDA decided to ask for evidence of safety. The FDA's decision to call for evidence after all that time is open to a number of political interpretations. Some believe that the manufacturers had a free ride during most of the 1980s because of the anti-regulatory philosophy of the Reagan administration. On the other hand, it is hard to escape the conclusion that the change in the FDA's attitude toward the end of the decade might also have reflected the mounting public concern about the issue, which in turn was largely driven by the publicity surrounding a few spectacular court cases. To the extent that this later interpretation is correct, the FDA responded like a political body, not a regulatory body.

In addition, after David Kessler came to the FDA in 1991, the controversy took on the character of a battle of wills. Kessler clearly believed in a strengthened FDA. The manufacturers, who had not performed the necessary studies to demonstrate safety, were cavalier in their response to the FDA's new hard line. Who would back down? Meanwhile, the public pressure to do something about breast implants was intensifying. Panels convened by the FDA to consider the matter included vocal partisans on the issue. Hearings were public and included emotional testimony about the harm caused by implants, but little critical analysis. The FDA's action, then, was taken in a charged atmosphere of advocacy and in the virtual absence of evidence. The ban raises the question of the degree to which regulatory decisions should be influenced by political and social considerations. It also raises the issue of the proper balance between regulatory protection of consumers and individual choice. In this case, the letter of the law, buttressed by public opinion, dictated one course, but consideration of the likely social consequences of a ban, particularly the widespread alarm, might have supported another.

The second theme illuminated by the breast implant story is the impact of tort law on American life. A tort is a wrongful act or injury for which damages are sought in a civil (as opposed to criminal) court. Americans increasingly turn to the courts to remedy a whole variety of complaints, and the number of tort cases—particularly product liability and malpractice cases—is growing accordingly. The breast implant case illustrates in the extreme the influence of the tort system. Even before the ban, there had been a steady trickle of lawsuits alleging that breast implants caused connective tissue or autoimmune disease. Successful lawsuits bred more lawsuits, which in turn bred publicity. Not surprisingly, as more women with implants and their doctors became aware of the possible risks, there were more reports of disease caused by implants. As the chairman of one of the FDA's panels said, "The lawyers were ahead of the doctors, and the public was ahead of the FDA."[11]

After the ban, the plaintiffs' bar moved quickly, and many thousands of lawsuits were filed within a matter of months. The result has been an immense transfer of money from the breast implant manufacturers to plaintiffs and their lawyers. There has been little attention to the fact that the money originates from consumers who purchase the manufacturers' other products. Nor has there been much attention to other consequences of the lawsuits, although they are likely to be far-reaching. In particular, manufacturers of other medical devices and the suppliers of their raw materials are threatening to pull out of the market because of the legal liabilities. What accounts for the torrent of successful litigation, with all its ripple effects, in the absence of solid scientific evidence about the risks of breast implants? Several peculiarities of the American tort system, which I will discuss in later chapters, bear on this question. Tort reform is now a contentious political issue, and the breast implant controversy throws the debate into sharp relief. It well exemplifies the tension between the pressure to curb the excesses of the tort system and the need to maintain reasonable access to the courts to seek redress for injury.

The third theme is the marginal and ambiguous role of scientific evidence in our society. To be sure, the United States has a large scientific enterprise, and its research findings are often widely publicized. But interest in scientific conclusions is not the same thing as interest in how they originated. The nature of evidence is simply not a front-burner item for most Americans, a fact illustrated by the breast implant story. As it happened, medical researchers did not systematically begin to collect evidence on breast implants until around the time of the FDA ban, when several large studies were initiated. These were epidemiologic studies that sought to determine whether the diseases said to be caused by breast implants are more common in women with implants than in women without implants. Unless this question is answered, it is impossible to say whether breast implants contribute to the diseases. Other types of studies, including animal studies, laboratory studies, and case reports, can raise interesting questions and answer some, but they cannot answer this one.

So far, none of the epidemiologic studies has been able to demonstrate a clear link between breast implants and connective tissue disease or suggestive symptoms. This does not mean that there cannot be a link, just that it is too small to have been detected by the studies that have been done. Possibly, much larger studies will show some risk. The answer to the question will come in incremental steps, one study at a time, and represent the accumulated weight of evidence from many sources. This is the way medical research works; evidence is accumulated slowly and the conclusion is inseparable from the evidence. The lack of understanding about how scientific conclusions are reached causes a great deal of confusion in American society, as I will discuss in a later chapter.

The fourth theme concerns science in the courtroom. When a trial involves a matter of scientific fact, such as whether breast implants cause disease, the approach to answering the question is very different in court than it is in scientific research. In the courtroom, expert witnesses, chosen and paid by the adversaries, are invited to give their opinion. The opinion may include some reference to research, published or unpublished, but it doesn't have to. If research is cited, there is no procedure for evaluating its reliability. Expert witnesses often simply refer vaguely to their "experience." What they are asked to provide, then, is essentially an educated guess. Although they are expected to have certain credentials, they needn't give the basis for their conclusions, except in the uncommon circumstance of a scientifically sophisticated cross-examination. This approach essentially reverses the scientific process. In science, the evidence leads to the conclusion; in the courtroom, the expert's conclusion comes first and *becomes* the legal evidence. Not surprisingly, the answers yielded by these two approaches may differ greatly.

Much of the discrepancy is simply a matter of how the legal process has been structured. But I believe it is exacerbated by a genuine lack of understanding between the two disciplines. The law and science represent two strikingly different ways of thinking, which reflect their different methods. The law frames questions in adversarial terms, and lawyers see problems as best resolved by controlled argument. In contrast, the scientific method is (ideally) not adversarial, but cooperative, and scientists usually find answers in the slow accumulation of evidence from many sources. The different ways of thinking are so ingrained that they may be virtually unconscious. For example, a lawyer questioning an epidemiologist in a deposition asked him why he was undertaking a study of breast implants when one had already been done. To the lawyer, a second study clearly implied that there was something wrong with the first. The epidemiologist was initially confused by the line of questioning. When he explained that no single study was conclusive, that all studies yielded tentative answers, that he was looking for consistency among a number of differently designed studies, it was the lawyer's turn to be confused. Similarly, I am occasionally asked by lawyers why the *New England Journal of Medicine* does not publish studies "on the other side," a concept that has no meaning in medical research. An adversarial approach is very effective for settling many types of disputes, which is no doubt why the law is based on it, but it is not the way to reach scientific conclusions. Yet science in the courtroom, no matter how inadequate, has great impact on people's lives and fortunes. Later I will discuss how the system might be reformed to make it better able to deal with scientific questions.

The fifth theme is the pervasive effect of the profit motive on so much of our public life. Just as the struggle to determine the *facts* about breast implants is between science and the law, the struggle for financial gain is between the manufacturers and the plaintiffs' attorneys. In their haste to cash in on the rapidly expanding market for silicone breast implants, the manufacturers glossed over their responsibility to perform adequate studies of the biological effects of implants. Internal memos from one manufacturer, Dow Corning, showed that there were safety concerns within the company that were not investigated. In fact, one memo instructed salespeople to wash the oily slick off implants before showing them to plastic surgeons at trade shows, thereby removing evidence of leakage. The overriding concern was to win the race against a competing manufacturer.

After the FDA ban, when the manufacturers were clearly on the ropes, the plaintiffs' attorneys moved in to capture the profits of the manufacturers. Since the lawyers are paid on a contingency basis—that is, a percentage of the plaintiff's award or out-of-court settlement—they had every interest in filing as many lawsuits as possible. If they lost most of them, it didn't matter. With contingency fees customarily in the range of 30 to 40 percent, all they needed was to win a few cases from time to time and settle most of them out of court. The system resulted in relatively small gains for many women and enormous gains for a few lawyers. The stake of the lawyers in the breast implant dispute is now so great that some of them have embarked on a campaign to discredit and harass scientists who are conducting epidemiologic research on the subject. Dr. Sherine Gabriel of the Mayo Clinic, author of the first published epidemiologic study of implants, was served with subpoenas demanding that she produce large numbers of documents about the women in her study. Authors of two other epidemiologic studies were served with similar subpoenas. These researchers say that responding to the subpoenas has been extremely burdensome and time-consuming. They believe the harassment might well dissuade other investigators from conducting epidemiologic studies. The avarice of manufacturers is necessarily restrained to some extent; if they are too obviously heedless of safety, they will lose their customers and find themselves in trouble with the law. Plaintiffs' attorneys are not similarly restrained. Their clients gain right along with them, and they are not only acting within the law, but using it as an instrument.

Finally, the sixth theme is the way in which the media present medical issues to the public. Until about 1990 the media had little to say about breast implants, except to report a few large jury verdicts. But as the time approached for the manufacturers to produce evidence of safety, the intermittent media reports became more frequent, until finally the media coverage was nearly incessant. It also grew more sensational and uncritical with time. On television and in newspapers and magazines, women—some of them celebrities—began to recount stories of deformity and disease stemming from their implants. The subject became a staple of talk shows. The tone of the coverage was anything but analytical. Instead, the premise that breast implants were dangerous seemed to be tacitly accepted. In addition, it was often strongly implied that the FDA, as well as the manufacturers, knew the devices were dangerous and suppressed the fact. The story played to both the American fascination with newly discovered, mass health hazards and the penchant to assume a cover-up in any disaster. Instead of presenting a complicated health story, the media simply generated outrage.

Which came first—the media spin or public opinion? As in all media-intensive stories, it is impossible to say because public opinion and media reports are so closely intertwined. What can be said is that the tone of the coverage almost certainly reflects a predisposition of the public to see it that way. The public is easily swept up in medical alarms, particularly when there is an element of wrongdoing involved. The power of the media and public opinion is immense, and that is by and large appropriate in a democracy. But not all endeavors are meant to be ruled by public opinion. Justice, for example, should not be, nor should science.

In subsequent chapters, I will consider each of the above themes using the breast implant controversy as a prism. But

first, it is necessary to review the nature of the implants themselves—how they were developed, what they are made of, how
the body reacts to them, and who has them and why. Understanding these devices makes it easier to see how the controversy about them illuminates the themes of this book.

2

BREAST IMPLANTS: WHAT THEY ARE AND WHO HAS THEM

I like a large casaba melon size, you know, I guess 40, 38.

—Unidentified man on CNN,
December 31, 1992

The female breast has always been a powerful symbol of femininity and sexuality, and the fact that women feel driven to have perfect breasts should be no surprise. Exactly what constitutes perfection changes with fashion. In the 1920s, women bound their breasts to make them look smaller. But over the following decades, until the waif look returned in the 1960s, women instead padded their bras to make their breasts look larger. After the anorectic look of the 1960s passed out of style and large breasts came into fashion again, padding had become a less feasible solution, since clothing was often too scanty to hide it. If breast size was to be increased, it had to be done from within. And that is what happened. During the 1970s, there was an explosion in the use of breast implants.[1] (Nevertheless, there is more than one way to be imperfect, and breast reduction surgery is almost as common as augmentation.)

In 1994 breast augmentation was the third most common cosmetic operation in the United States, despite the fact that the FDA ban had been in effect for almost two years.[2] Since implants filled with sterile saline (salt water) instead of silicone gel were allowed to remain on the market, women simply obtained them instead. The fee charged by surgeons was about $3,000. Only liposuction and eyelid surgery were more common. (Ironically, the same year, removing breast implants was the number-five procedure, no doubt reflecting the alarm following the FDA ban.) Breast augmentation is substantially more common in the Sunbelt—the southern and southwestern states and California—than it is elsewhere in the country.

At its peak, from 1979 to 1992, breast implant surgery was performed on about 100,000 to 150,000 American women each year. In today's dollars, this represented roughly $300 million to $450 million in surgical fees and $50 million to $75 million in manufacturers' revenues (assuming a price of $500 per set of implants). Although Dow Corning dominated the market, other manufacturers offered stiff competition: Bristol-Myers Squibb; Baxter International; Bioplasty, Inc.; Mentor Corporation; and McGhan Medical Corporation (now Inamed, once owned by the giant Minnesota Manufacturing and Mining Corporation [3M]). After the ban, of course, sales plummeted (Mentor stock fell from $30 in April 1991 to $8 in February 1992). Mentor and McGhan, the only manufacturers left in the market, continue to sell saline implants (about 40,000 of these are implanted each year). Mentor's silicone-gel-filled implants are offered for reconstruction only, and only under research conditions (about 22,000 yearly). Within months of the ban, the price of the saline implants had doubled and that of the silicone-gel-filled implants had tripled.[3]

Whether women reshape their breasts to please men or

to please themselves is a matter of debate. The distinction is difficult, because self-image is so bound up with the opinions of others. Women tend to interpret breast augmentation as a matter of self-image and enhanced confidence, while men tend to see it as a specific attempt to please them. For example, Arthur Caplan, a bioethicist at the University of Pennsylvania, in arguing that women do not have enough information to make an informed choice, told the *Boston Globe*, "I think having large breasts is an attempt to please males. It's a cultural fetish. American men are clearly enamored of mammary glands, and I'm all for giant boobs. But to invoke the language of choice is to invoke choice in a vacuum."[4] Some feminists, such as Naomi Wolf, author of *The Beauty Myth*, see the pressure on women to enlarge their breasts as more sinister. To Wolf, it is a way of stunting women's sexual capacity, as well as regimenting their appearance, since breast implant surgery sometimes decreases sensation in the nipples. Whether women get implants for themselves or to please men is not a meaningful question to her, since they do it within the context of a male-dominated society.[5]

The first known attempt to enlarge a woman's breasts occurred in Germany in 1895. (Interestingly, surgery to reduce breast size had been performed for many years.) In that first operation, fat from a benign tumor on the woman's back was transplanted to her breasts. Within a few years, surgeons were experimenting with paraffin wax to enlarge breasts. Later, other foreign substances were tried, including petroleum jelly, beeswax, and vegetable oils, but paraffin remained the mainstay. Probably the first women to turn to silicone were Japanese prostitutes after World War II, trying to satisfy the taste of American occupation forces for Western-style large breasts. Instead of having discrete packets of silicone surgically implanted in their breasts, as is now done, these women had liquid silicone or paraffin injected by needle or tube directly into their breast tissue, often along with assorted contaminants. Within a few years, breast augmentation by silicone injection had spread to the United States, where it found particular favor among Las Vegas showgirls and aspiring actresses in California.[6]

Silicone seemed like the perfect substance to enlarge breasts. It is made by stringing together silicon and oxygen, the two most common elements of the earth's crust, and adding organic groups to form chains or polymers. Depending on the length and configuration of the polymer, the silicone can have nearly any consistency, including liquid, gel, or rubbery solid (elastomer). First synthesized just before World War II, silicone came into widespread use during the war for insulation, lubrication, and sealing. In addition, it found almost immediate use in medicine because of its remarkable inertness in the human body. It does not degrade appreciably, it is highly resistant to bacterial contamination, and living tissues seem to accept it readily.[7] For these reasons, silicone is a component of artificial joints and heart valves, shunts and other tubings, disposable needles and syringes, and contraceptive implants (Norplant), as well as testicular and penile implants. Indeed, probably no American is without some silicone in his or her body, put there by some type of routine medical care—such as injections with silicone-lubricated needles and syringes. But despite its special properties and seeming safety, injecting a large volume of liquid silicone of uncertain purity directly into the breasts led to serious problems.

Any foreign substance or object introduced into the body's tissues provokes an inflammatory response. It is necessary to have a general idea of the inflammatory response to understand the breast implant controversy fully. Consider a splinter, which is a foreign object. If a splinter is left under the skin, even if it isn't carrying bacteria, the area will become slightly reddened and swollen because of an increased blood flow carrying large numbers of special cells to the area. The function of these cells—called white cells—is to try to engulf, break down, and dissolve the foreign object. It is an attempt by the body to get rid of something that doesn't belong there. Eventually, if the foreign object remains in the body, most of the white cells are replaced with fibrous scar tissue, which consists mainly of microscopic fibers made of a firm substance called collagen.

The increased blood flow and gathering of white cells is termed inflammation. When inflammation is a response to a foreign object, like a splinter, it is called a "foreign-body reaction." The process can be mild or intense, depending on the nature of the foreign object, the location in the body, and the particular individual's reactivity. If the object is contaminated with bacteria, the inflammation is likely to be severe and ongoing. White cells will keep entering the area to battle the infection, even while scar tissue is forming. When you have a dirty splinter, for example, the area is very much redder and more swollen than is the case with a clean one. Sometimes pus forms, which is simply tissue fluid containing enormous numbers of dead white cells. When the foreign body is sterile, as is the case with breast implants, the inflammation is replaced by scar tissue. With time all scar tissue contracts and becomes firm. (If you have a surgical scar, say, from an appendectomy, you will know exactly what I mean. First the scar is pink and raised; later it becomes smaller and white, and may even become depressed below the level of the surrounding skin as it contracts.) Scar tissue in the breast is no exception. As it would anywhere else, it becomes firm with time and tends to contract. This contracture has great significance in the breast implant controversy, as we will see.

In general, silicone elicits only a very mild inflammatory response. But when large amounts of liquid silicone were injected directly into the breast, as was done to the Japanese prostitutes, there were often terrible consequences. Bacterial contamination from dirty needles or contaminated silicone was common. It wasn't just silicone that was being injected, but all manner of other substances and bacteria. A severe inflammatory reaction often formed around each tiny globule of silicone, making the breasts lumpy and hard, particularly as the scar tissue contracted. Because the liquid silicone tended to migrate into the soft tissues around the breasts or in the armpits, it was customary to add irritating substances, such as olive oil, so that there would be even more scar tissue to trap the silicone and anchor it in place. The scarring around silicone globules could then become so severe that it produced grotesque lumps that resembled tumors. In addition, when the breasts became infected, gangrenous sores sometimes developed on the overlying skin or nipple. Needless to say, besides being disfiguring, the complications of directly injecting silicone were often excruciatingly painful.[8]

BY THE EARLY 1960S the problems with injecting liquid silicone into the breasts were all too apparent. For a while, there had been attempts to augment breasts by implanting sponges made of polyvinyl alcohol, rather than by injecting silicone, but there were problems with this method, too. The scar tissue that formed around each sponge also filled all the little holes in it. Thus, when the scar contracted, it squeezed the sponge into a small, hard ball.[9]

In 1961, two Houston plastic surgeons, Thomas Cronin and Frank Gerow, began work on a different sort of implantable device.[10] It is said that Gerow was inspired by the similarity between the consistency of a plastic transfusion bag containing blood and the feel of a breast. Whatever his inspiration, Gerow visited Dow Corning, then the leading manufacturer of silicone, to suggest that they collaborate in designing a breast implant made of silicone. Dow Corning, which was formed by Dow Chemical and Corning Glass Works to take advantage of the burgeoning silicone market after World War II, was at that time in the process of developing its Medical Products Division. The following year, 1962, Gerow placed the first modern breast implants (Dow Corning's Silastic mammary prosthesis) in a woman who wanted to enlarge her breasts. (Now a sixty-four-year-old grandmother, she still has her original implants today and professes to be content with them.) The implants consisted of a rubbery silicone envelope containing silicone gel. Packaging the silicone in this way was intended to eliminate migration, as well as the irritating effects of large liquid injections. This is still the basic design of breast implants, which look like smooth, soft plastic bags of various shapes, containing about a cup of clear jelly. In the early years they often had Dacron patches attached to the back to generate more scar tissue to hold them in place, but that feature was later abandoned.

Placement of the implants is remarkably simple. It requires only two small incisions, usually in the crease under each breast, although sometimes the incisions are made around the nipples. Through the incision, the surgeon creates a pocket behind the breast tissue and squeezes the implant into it, so that it lies behind the breast and in front of the underlying muscle. From this position, the implant pushes forward the natural breast tissue.[11] The procedure is somewhat more difficult in women who are getting implants for reconstruction after mastectomy for breast cancer. In these cases, the implant is usually not placed in front of the muscle, because, with the breast gone, it would be too close to the skin and might actually rub through it. Instead, it is placed either behind the muscle, against the ribs, or between layers of the muscle. Sometimes reconstruction is done at the time of the mastectomy; sometimes there is a delay of a few months, until the mastectomy has healed. A nipple is usually reconstructed from skin or mucous membranes taken from elsewhere on the body.[12]

The gel-filled implants were almost immediately seen to be a great improvement over direct injections, and they quickly became the favored method of augmentation. They looked and felt natural, they were sterile, and they did not migrate. Nevertheless, at least four problems became apparent almost from the beginning: contractures from scarring, leakage of silicone, rupture, and difficulties in performing mammography.[13] The major one was the scarring that inevitably occurred around the implant envelope as a result of the foreign-body reaction. This was not as extreme as the scarring around globules of injected silicone, but it was still the same basic process. In the case of implants, the fibrous scar tissue formed all around each implant, encasing it in a "capsule." In and of itself, the capsule was not a problem. It was usually not very thick and it was, of course, invisible. The problem came as the scar tissue contracted. The capsule would then squeeze the implant, making it hard and unnaturally rounded. Severe contractures produced visible bulges in the upper part of the breasts, which were often painful. No one knows what percentage of women with breast implants suffer from noticeable contractures, but it is probably a substantial fraction, perhaps as many as half. Nor is it clear why some women are more susceptible to this problem than others.

In the 1970s a second problem was discovered. It became apparent that small quantities of silicone fluid from the gel leaked through the envelope, even though the envelope was intact. This slow leakage is called "bleeding" or "sweating," and it seems to be caused by tiny molecules of the gel migrating through the pores in the surrounding envelope. Women are not aware of the silicone leakage, because it is so slow and the amounts are so small. Nevertheless, it has been a cause for great concern, because silicone thereby escapes into the body. Usually the leakage is contained within the encasing capsule of scar tissue, but sometimes tiny particles of silicone can be found in nearby lymph glands. Whether the leakage contributes to the thickness of the capsule by exacerbating the inflammatory process is not known, but it is a reasonable conjecture.

For years surgeons would try to relieve excessive contracture by a procedure known as a "closed capsulotomy"—forcefully squeezing the breast by hand to rupture the scar tissue.[14] The trouble with closed capsulotomy is that it not only ruptures the capsule, but often ruptures the envelope of the implant as well, causing the sudden release of silicone gel into the tissues, unimpeded by the presence of an intact capsule. When this happens, small amounts of silicone may be engulfed by white cells and transported through the lymphatic system to distant parts of the body. In addition to the risk of rupture, capsulotomy often causes acute inflammation (mastitis) from the trauma to the tissues (forcefully squeezing the breasts is not easy on them). Even when closed capsulotomy did not cause rupture of the envelope, it was often only partially successful, so that the implant bulged out on one side. And in any case the scar tissue almost always re-formed.[15] Most plastic surgeons no longer perform the procedure, although it was once extremely common. By 1980 Dow Corning included in its package insert a warning against closed capsulotomy, which concluded, "Such abnormal trauma or stress to the breasts could result in prosthesis rupture with extravasation of gel into surrounding tissue." All this means is: Squeeze the breast implants too hard and they will burst.

When an implant and its capsule rupture suddenly, whether from a closed capsulotomy or a blow to the chest, the breast loses its shape as the silicone escapes into the tissues. Often, however, there is only a small tear, and the escaping silicone gel remains trapped within the capsule. In this case, the woman may not be aware that she has a rupture. The exact incidence of rupture that is noticed by the woman remains unknown. The manufacturers have estimated a rate of 1 percent or less, but others estimate it to be higher, closer to 5 percent. The incidence of slight rupture that is unnoticed and contained within the capsule is even more difficult to determine. One study found unappreciated rupture in 5 percent of women with implants who were having mammograms.[16]

Difficulty in performing mammography is a fourth problem. It is not exactly a complication, but a necessary concomitant of having breast implants. The difficulty stems from the fact that the implant obstructs the passage of x-rays through the breast tissue. Whether this problem has resulted in cancer being diagnosed later in its course is not clear. What is clear is that mammography in women with implants requires more care. The implant must be manipulated so that it is held against the chest wall, while the breast tissue is pulled away from it. Multiple views may be required. The technical problems in performing mammography are occasionally confused with the issue of whether the implants themselves increase the risk of cancer. There is no evidence that they do. At first, Dow Corning had the breast implant market to itself, but later other manufacturers began to make implants and the market became very competitive. Innovations followed rapidly, most of them designed to counter the twin problems of contractures and leakage. One such innovation, designed to reduce the tendency of the capsule to harden and contract, was to coat the outside of the implants with polyurethane foam. Because of the fuzzy texture of these implants, the scar tissue that formed around them was more irregular than the capsules that form around smooth implants. It was thought that the irregularity would make strong contractures less likely, because the scar tissue would not all be pulling in the same direction. At first the idea seemed to work. The breasts remained softer than with the smooth-textured implants—at least for the first few months. But eventually the contractures became just as bad, as a thick, regular capsule formed around the initial irregular one. Furthermore, the polyurethane-coated implants were extremely difficult to remove because there was no well-defined capsule to demarcate them. They were all bound up in the breast tissue, with no clear boundary. In addition, some women with polyurethane-coated implants developed an angry, red rash on the skin over the breasts.[17]

Another innovation was designed to deal with the silicone leakage problem by filling the envelope with sterile saline instead of silicone gel. The leakage would then consist not of silicone, but saline, which is known to be harmless. The problem with saline-filled implants is that their consistency is not as natural as gel-filled implants. To deal with the unnatural consistency, manufacturers tried using a double envelope, yielding two compartments, one inside the other. The inner one contained silicone gel and the outer one contained saline. The purpose was to limit the bleeding of the silicone through the outer envelope by enclosing it in a layer of saline. The double-envelope implants were banned along with ordinary silicone-gel-filled implants in 1992. The single-envelope saline implants have another problem, in addition to their relatively unnatural consistency. Unlike silicone-gel-filled implants, they are not pre-filled. Instead, the surgeon places the empty silicone envelopes behind the breasts, then fills them with sterile saline through a valve. If the envelopes are overfilled, they are too hard; if they are underfilled, they crumple and cause wrinkles in the skin above them. Furthermore, saline-filled implants sometimes spontaneously empty. For all these reasons, they have not been as popular as silicone-gel-filled implants.[18]

Before the FDA ban about 97 percent of women who had implants chose ones filled with silicone gel. A little over half were smooth textured; most of the remainder were polyurethane coated.[19] Now, of course, only saline-filled implants are generally available, so by default they are being used a great deal more. Eventually, however, their manufacturers will have to submit evidence of their safety to the FDA to keep them on the market. The most recent innovation is to fill the silicone envelope with soybean oil, which, unlike silicone and saline, is translucent to mammography. Not only would these not interfere with mammography, but it is hoped that the soybean oil would be innocuous if released into the tissues after rupture. They, too, will require FDA approval.[20]

RUMORS that this or that movie star had silicone injections or implants have circulated freely since the 1950s, when Marilyn

Monroe and Jayne Mansfield set a very tough standard for the female form—as Dolly Parton does now. But despite the rumors, celebrities have in general kept the matter private, as have most other women. Only in the last decade or so have women, usually in court, been willing to tell of their efforts to enlarge and reshape their breasts. One of the first celebrities to go directly to the public with her breast implant story was Jenny Jones, the TV talk show host. Jones, who projects a persona of sweet vulnerability, told her story to *People* magazine, as well as twice on her talk show. She said she had been through five sets of implants, each of which caused rock-like hardening and distortion of her breasts. She had dutifully kneaded and squeezed her breasts, as advised by her plastic surgeon, in an attempt to soften and reshape them, despite the fact that at least some manufacturers warned in the package inserts that this could cause rupture. Because she had the polyurethane-coated implants (and over the years a few of her implants had ruptured), removing them was extremely difficult. Jones's highly public revelations came at the time David Kessler, with much attendant publicity, was trying to decide whether to ban implants.

Why had Jones put herself through all this? She told *People* that as a young woman she had suffered because she was flat-chested. "I would look at sexy nightgowns and lingerie," she said, "and think that I could never wear them." In 1981 she sold nearly everything she owned (she was poorer then) to pay for breast implants. This was shortly after her divorce, and the timing was evidently not coincidental. As she explained, "My husband seldom touched my breasts when we were intimate. I could only assume that they were not big enough or attractive enough for him." She also told of surveying the men on her staff "about what makes a woman sexy, and the number one thing on almost every sheet was big boobs—big breasts." I am skeptical that most men would subscribe to this ranking, but still, it's generally assumed that men prefer large breasts. Appearances are very important in the mating game, and the mating game is very important to most of us. Jenny Jones showed us just how desperate the whole thing could get.[21]

The actress Mariel Hemingway also spoke frankly about her experience with breast implants. She got silicone-gel-filled breast implants when she was eighteen years old and had been chosen to play a *Playboy* centerfold in the film *Star 80*. She said of her decision to get implants, "I didn't do it for the movie, I did it for myself. I don't like to talk about it much, but yeah, it gave me self-esteem. It made me feel like a girl, and I had never felt like a girl. I always felt like this tall thing." After the FDA ban, she was concerned enough to have her silicone implants removed and replaced by saline implants, which, incidentally, were smaller. A year later, now thirty-two and married, she was ready to do without implants altogether. As she put it, "I'm a woman now. I'm married and have two kids. I don't need those things."[22]

Over the three decades that silicone breast implants were freely available, there were marked changes in the pattern of their use. Initially, like silicone injections, they were a tool of the trade for showgirls and aspiring actresses. For them, the bigger the breasts, the better for business. They wanted unnaturally large implants to please their male audiences. Ordinary women were both envious and appalled. They did not immediately rush to emulate women with breast implants. But with time, women began to see breast implants as a way to improve their figures, without necessarily seeking to have "casaba melon size" breasts. Manufacturers responded by producing

implants of various sizes and shapes, including less protuber-
ant ones, known as "low-profile" implants, and implants with
round, oval, and teardrop shapes. By 1992, about 1 percent of
American women had breast implants—with enticing names
like Misti-Gold, Même, Natural-Y, and Replicon.

The pattern of breast implant use in Olmsted County,
Minnesota, the location of the Mayo Clinic (and a conserva-
tive, rural midwestern community), is illuminating. Breast implant surgery there increased rapidly from 1964 to 1979.
Whereas in 1964 there were only 3.5 implant recipients per
100,000 population, in 1979 there were 95 per 100,000. After
that initial burst, the use stabilized. As a fraction of the total,
women who had implants for reconstruction after breast cancer surgery grew from 10 percent in 1964 to 30 percent in
1991, and the average age of implant recipients increased
from twenty-eight to thirty-six. Over time there was also a
much greater variability in ages, with both much younger and
much older women receiving them. Initially, only married
women in Olmsted County got implants; in 1991 about 15 percent were single. Although breast implant use is substantially
greater in some other parts of the country, the *pattern* of use
in Olmsted County is probably fairly representative of the rest
of the country. Unfortunately, we simply do not have very
good information on the subject. A smaller survey of women
who had implants for augmentation showed an average age
of thirty-eight; just over half were married. As in other surveys,
women with breast implants were relatively well-educated and
affluent.[23]

After the early years, most women who had breast implants no longer wanted to be conspicuous, but rather to fit
in—to feel more normal. A 1990 survey commissioned by the
American Society of Plastic and Reconstructive Surgeons

found the most common reason given was to achieve better body proportions.[24] Many women claim that the devices have greatly increased their confidence and their enjoyment of life. Even when there are local complications, as there frequently are, these women do not want to lose their implants. When severe contractures develop or an implant ruptures, many women simply replace the implants with new ones. To them, the complications are simply an annoyance, and well worth the benefits. But others feel equally strongly that breast implants are an affront to women's dignity, and that those who acquire them for augmentation have been victimized. As Jones said, "If it was perfectly safe, there is still a bigger issue. Small breasts are not the problem. It's how harshly we judge ourselves and how we judge each other." To these women, any risk, no matter how small, is too high a price to pay for a procedure that is so self-abnegating.

Whatever the cultural meanings, most women with cosmetic implants are pleased with them. The 1990 survey mentioned above found that over 90 percent were satisfied with them and would make the same choice again. However, in a very small survey taken in 1991, as the controversy about safety became more intense, only 60 percent said they were satisfied and nearly 40 percent said they had experienced complications, principally contractures, although some complained also of decreased sensation in the breasts or nipples. Still, only about 10 percent said they were so dissatisfied that they regretted having the implants and only 6 percent planned to have them removed.[25] It is hard to interpret the answers to polls and surveys, particularly when the samples are very small. Nevertheless, there seems to be a good deal of ambivalence about breast implants, as evidenced by the fact that the vast majority of women who have them do not regret their decision, yet about a third have registered for a class-action settlement based on the premise that implants are risky. Many women seem to be simultaneously satisfied and apprehensive.

The debate about the meaning of breast implants for women, whether they are exploitative or enhancing, leaves open the question of exactly what the risk is. The FDA was supposedly not taking a sociologic stand, but a regulatory one. Why did it ban silicone-gel-filled breast implants? The next chapter addresses that question.

3

THE FDA BAN ON IMPLANTS: REGULATION IN MODERN AMERICA

Caveat emptor has never been—and never will be—the philosophy at the FDA.

—David Kessler, Chairman of the FDA,
June 18, 1992

In November 1990, when President George Bush appointed David Kessler as commissioner of the FDA, the Republican president, presumably no proponent of government regulation, was choosing someone utterly committed to the spirit as well as the letter of the law of regulating drugs and devices. Bush was also choosing someone with apparently superhuman energy. Kessler, an intense, wiry man in his forties, with thick glasses and a trim carrot-colored beard and mustache, has a medical degree from Harvard and a law degree from the University of Chicago, obtained nearly simultaneously while he commuted between Boston and Chicago. He then trained in pediatrics at Johns Hopkins Medical School, while serving as a consultant to Senator Orrin Hatch (R-Utah). (His commute was then down to the distance between Baltimore and Washington.) Later Kessler became medical director of the Albert Einstein Hospital in New York City, but here again one full-time job was not enough. He also taught food and drug law at Columbia Law School, and obtained an advanced professional certificate from New York University's Graduate School of Business Administration. Upon being appointed commissioner of the FDA, he threw himself into the job with his customary drive and with a zeal not seen in earlier commissioners.[1]

When Kessler arrived in Washington, breast implants had been on the market for nearly 30 years, but they had been under the purview of the FDA only since 1976. That year the Medical Device Amendment to the Food, Drug, and Cosmetic Act extended the FDA's authority to cover devices, as well as food, drugs, and cosmetics. Under this amendment, manufacturers of new devices could, at the discretion of the FDA, be required to submit an application for premarketing approval. The applications were to include data on safety and effectiveness from animal and human studies. Until FDA approval was obtained, new devices that required premarketing approval could not be sold. Since breast implants were already on the market, they were "grandfathered" (exempted because they predated the amendment), at least for the time being. Presumably, given their long track record, they were reasonably safe. Nevertheless, in 1982 the FDA proposed requiring "premarketing approval," which meant the manufacturers would have to supply evidence of the safety of implants.[2]

The FDA did nothing more about breast implants until 1988, when it finalized the 1982 proposal. This action came in the wake of the first few anecdotal reports in medical journals of cases of connective tissue disease in women who had undergone breast augmentation. The earliest reports emanated from Japan and concerned directly injected paraffin or silicone, not implants.[3] In 1982, however, an Australian physician reported connective tissue disease in three women who had silicone-gel-filled implants.[4] The FDA's action was undoubtedly also influenced by successful lawsuits in the United States that followed the 1982 report. The first of these, the 1984 case of Maria Stern, resulted in a jury award of nearly $2 million.[5] When the FDA in 1988 asked for evidence of safety and effectiveness, the manufacturers were by law given at least 30 months to gather the data. Despite the extended time, producing the evidence was a daunting task and one the manufacturers no doubt resented, since they had enjoyed being grandfathered for so many years.

Events then began to move rapidly, driven largely by a small number of people who happened to be in the right place at the right time. One was Dan Bolton, a young plaintiffs' attorney in San Francisco, whose firm handled the case of Maria Stern. In preparing for the trial, Bolton, then fresh out of Hastings Law School, was sent by his firm (Hersh and Hersh) to the Dow Corning plant in Midland, Michigan, to see what he could learn (a legal process called "discovery"). There he found a number of internal documents that, according to Bolton, indicated the implants were known by the company to be unsafe. After the verdict in the Stern case, a settlement was reached that included "sealing" the documents—that is, forbidding them to be made public. Much was later made of these "secret documents," and I will come back to them.[6] Another influential player was Dr. Norman Anderson, associate professor of medicine and surgery at Johns Hopkins Medical School. Anderson was the chairman of a 1988 FDA advisory panel that was convened to consider what safety data the manufacturers would be required to supply. He apparently became convinced early on that the implants were dangerous, perhaps partly influenced by Bolton, who testified before the 1988 panel.[7] As the controversy heated up, Anderson seemed to turn up everywhere.

Ralph Nader's consumer group, Public Citizen, also became involved early. The director of its Health Research Group, Dr. Sidney Wolfe, in 1988 petitioned former FDA commissioner Frank Young (who preceded Kessler in the position) to ban breast implants and scolded him in a letter for taking so long to demand assurances of safety: "You must explain why six and one-half years elapsed before finalizing the FDA's January 19, 1982, proposal to require Dow and other companies making silicone gel breast implants to submit safety data. Your agency negligently did not finalize this regulation until June of this year."[8] Bolton, Anderson, and Wolfe often reinforced one another's efforts. Bolton, for example, began to assist other plaintiffs' attorneys through Public Citizen's breast implant clearinghouse.[9] Another influential player was Sybil Goldrich, co-founder of an advocacy group called Command Trust Network, devoted largely to referring women with implants to plaintiffs' attorneys. Goldrich is herself a survivor of breast cancer who received breast implants for reconstruction. She has been indefatigable in her campaign against implants, and her organization is well connected with a number of highly successful plaintiffs' attorneys specializing in breast implant cases.[10]

Perhaps the most important event to bring the growing unease about breast implants to the attention of the public was Connie Chung's sensational treatment of the matter in 1990. On her TV show, *Face to Face with Connie Chung,* she conveyed the clear message that implants were dangerous devices foisted off on unsuspecting women. Introducing the segment with, "Coming up, some shocking information about breast implants," Chung interviewed women who claimed they had autoimmune disease caused by breast implants. Without questioning the presumed link between the disease and the implants, Chung implicitly blamed the FDA for permitting such risky products to be sold.[11] At about the same time, the late congressman Ted Weiss (D-N.Y.), chair of the Human Resources Subcommittee (which oversees the FDA), held hearings on the subject. In his testimony before the Weiss subcommittee, Anderson said, "Despite estimates that 2 million women bear these devices, we cannot even quantitate the short-term risks for these consumers." Less restrained was Sybil Goldrich, who testified, "I've gone seven years without a recurrence of cancer but what will happen from the silicone? I shudder when I think about it."[12] Consumers were well mobilized. What remained was for David Kessler to act.

When Kessler took over the FDA in 1991, the manufacturers had not yet responded to the FDA's 1988 order to present data on safety and effectiveness. On April 10, 1991, Kessler notified the manufacturers that there was to be no more delay. They had 90 days to file their premarketing applications.[13] Almost immediately, Bristol-Myers Squibb's Surgitek Corporation, manufacturer of the polyurethane-coated implants, withdrew them from the market, ostensibly because the foam degraded into toluene diamine, known to be a carcinogen in animals.[14] When the deadline arrived, only four of the major manufacturers—Mentor Corporation, McGhan Medical Corporation, Dow Corning Corporation, and Bioplasty, Inc.— even bothered to complete premarketing applications, and these were clearly inadequate. The FDA asked for more and better data.[15] In November 1991, it convened another advisory panel, this time chaired by Dr. Elizabeth Connell, professor of gynecology and obstetrics at Emory University Medical

School, although Norman Anderson was again a member. The public meeting featured heated testimony and attracted considerable publicity. Such venerable mainstream groups as the AMA and the American Cancer Society, as well as, not surprisingly, the American Society of Plastic and Reconstructive Surgeons, favored leaving the implants on the market. But they were up against determined consumer and advocacy groups and, most important, a series of women who recounted poignant stories of the suffering they had endured as a result of their implants. The panel concluded that the manufacturers had failed to provide reasonable assurances of the safety and effectiveness of silicone-gel implants. Calling the lack of data "appalling," they suggested that the manufacturers gather more and better evidence over the next year or two. Despite the dereliction of the manufacturers, however, the panel unanimously recommended that the devices be permitted to remain on the market. In the panel's view, they clearly filled a consumer need and there was no reason to believe they were unsafe. Kessler said he would make his decision over the next month or two, but it was expected that he would follow his panel's recommendation and leave the implants on the market.[16]

Just a month later, on December 13, 1991, a federal jury in San Francisco awarded what was then the largest verdict ever in a breast implant case—$7.34 million.[17] The plaintiff, Mariann Hopkins, claimed her implants had caused her to develop a rare disorder—mixed connective tissue disease. She was represented by none other than Dan Bolton, whom she had decided to retain after seeing him on television.[18] In the trial, Bolton made much of the secret documents he had found at the Dow Corning plant nine years earlier, while preparing for the Stern case.[19] After the walloping verdict in the Hopkins case, which I will describe in more detail later, Anderson and Bolton both urgently pressed Kessler to ban the implants, at least until the FDA could review the secret documents.[20] Kessler responded by demanding the documents and sending FDA investigators to Dow Corning to search their records. In January 1992, instead of making a final decision, Kessler called for a temporary moratorium on breast implants while he considered the matter further. He explained that he had come into possession of new information that compelled him to take another look. "We cannot assure the safety of this product," said Kessler, and he reconvened his advisory panel to consider the new evidence. In the meantime, in response to FDA pressure, Dow Corning released 800 pages of the notorious documents on February 10, 1992.[21]

When the advisory panel met again, on February 18, 1992, again in open session, the publicity was even more intense than it had been in November. Anderson had been stripped of his vote, an action the FDA said was "necessitated by statements in the mass media which led to an appearance of his inability to render objective advice." Still, he was permitted to stay on the panel as a nonvoting member, and the FDA openly acknowledged that he had been instrumental in getting them to take another look at the manufacturers' activities. (Later Anderson claimed that Kessler was "moving forward to leave silicone breast implants on the market," and had reversed himself only when Anderson presented him with Dow Corning's secret documents.[22])

In the end, after a good deal of impassioned testimony, the panel recommended that silicone-gel-filled breast implants be removed from the market, except under stringently limited conditions. They could be used only as a part of cancer treatment for women who agree to participate in research studies and, possibly in the future, in research studies of a very small number of healthy women receiving implants for breast augmentation. Kessler accepted this recommendation, and on April 16, 1992, announced the virtual ban of silicone-gel-filled breast implants.[23] (It was after the panel's February meeting and before Kessler's final action that Jenny Jones told her story on television. One of her guests was Norman Anderson, who at the close of the show said of her crusade against breast implants, "Jenny, you've started a national leadership whether you like it or not." Anderson himself was no bit player.)

WHILE THE NOOSE TIGHTENED, breast implant manufacturers fought a rear-guard action, with one eye on their markets and the other on their regulatory and legal problems. Thus, they were in the odd position of arguing simultaneously that breast implants were not associated with connective tissue diseases, but, even if they were, the manufacturers had duly warned their customers. After the success of the first lawsuit alleging such a connection (the 1984 Stern case), Dow Corning had acknowledged in its package inserts "reports of suspected immunological responses to silicone mammary implants," but added, "A review of the published experimental findings and clinical experience shows that convincing evidence does not exist to support a causal relationship between exposure to silicone materials and the acquisition or exacerbation of a variety of rheumatic and connective tissue disorders."[24] The company was right about the lack of evidence that the implants were dangerous. But there was also little evidence that they were safe, because the manufacturers had not fulfilled their responsibility to look for it.

As for the much ballyhooed "secret documents," they turned out to be a mix of things: an assortment of internal memos and minutes of meetings of Dow Corning employees; records of animal testing dating back to the 1960s; calculations of leakage rates and other physical properties of the implants; complaints from plastic surgeons, mainly concerning leakage or rupture; and accounts of ruptured implants returned to the company. The animal studies were fairly extensive, but mostly involved the direct injection of various forms of silicone into different parts of the animals' bodies. Some of these suggested that silicone could be carried from one part of the body to another. Only a few studies simulated the use of implants in women by placing similar devices in animals. One of these, a study of four dogs, received a great deal of attention because the documents showed there was chronic inflammation around the implants. Was this evidence of an immune reaction, as many critics assert, or was it merely a local, nonspecific response, as Dow Corning maintains? The documents also referred to rats developing sarcomas in response to injected silicone, but Dow Corning's accompanying explanatory material pointed out that sarcomas are common in rats in response to nearly any irritant. In contrast, this type of tumor is rare in humans and almost never occurs in human breast tissue. The significance of all this was, and still is, unclear, since the experiments had little in common with the ordinary use of breast implants in women.

Perhaps the most incriminating of the "secret documents" were the memos and minutes of meetings of a Mammary Task Force formed in 1975 to develop a new, softer gel to give the implants a more natural consistency. Headed by Arthur Rathjen, this task force was clearly under great pressure to bring a new product to market by an established deadline (Rathjen's minutes of meetings usually included the number of weeks, days, hours, and minutes left). There was concern in the task force that the new, softer gel might tend to leak through the envelope more than the firmer gel. As it turned out, the data showed the leakage to be somewhat less, but there was reason for the concern. The Dow Corning salespeople were finding that plastic surgeons to whom they showed the new implants complained that there was an oily coating on the surface of the envelope. In response, a member of the task force wrote the following memo to the salespeople:

> It has been observed that the new mammaries with responsive gel have a tendency to appear oily after being manipulated. This could prove to be a problem with your daily detailing activity where mammary manipulation is a must. Keep in mind that this is not a product problem; our technical people assure us that the doctor in the O. R. will not see any appreciable oiling on product removed from the package. The oily phenomenon seems to appear the day following manipulation. You should make plans to change demonstration samples often. Also, be sure samples are clean and dry before customer detailing. Two easy ways to clean demonstration samples while traveling, 1) wash with soap and water in nearest washroom, dry with hand towels, 2) carry a small bottle of IPA and rag. I have used both methods and the first is my choice. I will be interested to hear if any of you are seeing the oiling.

This obviously duplicitous memo would come back to haunt Dow Corning again and again. It showed unequivocally that Dow Corning was willing to hide evidence that silicone fluid leaked through the envelope.

The "secret documents" also showed that key employees were well aware of how little Dow Corning knew about their implants, and they anticipated the sorts of questions they would need to address. Rathjen wrote in 1976, "We better get going on a basic long-range project relative to gel, its formulation, toxicology, etc., over and above what is now underway." And more excitedly, "Is there something in the implant that migrates out or off the mammary prosthesis? Yes or no! Does it continue for the life of the implant, or is it limited or controlled for a period of time? Does it come from the gel, or envelope, or both? What is it?"

But the secret documents, revealing as they were, did not yield a smoking gun. They did not show a clear risk that the company had suppressed. Whether leakage, inflammation, capsule formation, or rupture could be dangerous to women was simply not systematically studied. What the documents did indicate was how little was known, how inadequate the studies had been, and how relentlessly the company pursued its market goals.[25] Adding to Dow Corning's problems was the discovery in 1992 that employees falsified some of the data about the manufacturing process, a charge that Dow Corning admitted. Evidently, some of the employees doctored the the automatic recordings of failures in the heat-curing process for the implants. According to Dow Corning, they did it to avoid the review they would undergo if the failures were faithfully recorded.[26]

Dow Corning pulled out of the implant market the month before Kessler's final decision.[27] Only two American manufacturers remained in the implant business—Mentor Corporation and McGhan(now Inamed). Mentor was granted approval to begin clinical studies of silicone implants used for reconstruction.[28] McGhan's saline implants were left on the market, as were Mentor's, but in 1993 the FDA announced that saline implants, too, would be subject retroactively to a premarketing application,[29] as would testicular prostheses.[30] (The fate of the latter will surely test the view that women are treated differently than men by the FDA.)

KESSLER IS KNOWN to be a man of strong opinions, and this, along with his combative style, perhaps belied the extent to which he was pressured by a variety of forces, most notably by aggrieved breast implant recipients and various advocacy groups. In view of the paucity of evidence of risk, Kessler knew that the scientific community would be critical of a ban on implants. Perhaps for this reason, he undertook to defend the ban vigorously, most clearly in a 1992 article in the *New England Journal of Medicine*. In it he acknowledged that his decision "was one of the most controversial decisions ever made by the agency," given the lack of evidence about safety and the intense feelings on both sides. But, he said, "the burden of proof rests squarely with the manufacturer." According to the law, Kessler said, the FDA did not have to show that breast implants were unsafe; the manufacturers had to show they were safe. As for a woman's choice, Kessler said, "It has become fashionable in some quarters to argue that women ought to be able to make such decisions on their own. If members of our society were empowered to make their own decisions about the entire range of products for which the FDA has responsibility, however, then the whole rationale for the agency would cease to exist." And more grandly, in that pre-Gingrich era, "Caveat emptor has never been—and never will be—the philosophy at the FDA."[31]

I had doubts that the matter was as clear-cut as Kessler implied. In an editorial in the same issue of the *New England Jour-*

nal of Medicine, I pointed out that all drugs and devices carry risks of side effects, sometimes quite serious ones. The FDA had never demanded that a drug or device be risk-free, only that the risks be commensurate with the benefits. The greater the potential benefits, the greater the acceptable risks. The job of the FDA, I pointed out, is to gather information on both benefits and risks, and balance them. If the balance is reasonable (a necessarily imprecise judgment), then the drug or device should be approved.[32] But in the case of breast implants, there were special problems. First, as Kessler emphasized, we didn't know enough about possible risks. He was careful to say that this didn't mean that implants were dangerous, only that we did not have sufficient information to know one way or the other. Our ignorance was not total, of course. We had, after all, 30 years of experience with breast implants in 1 million to 2 million women, and this was why breast implants had been grandfathered in the first place. We knew that the great majority of women with implants were satisfied with them. As already noted, we also knew that in about 5 percent of women, implants ruptured and had to be replaced, and that there was hardening of the breasts in many more women (although not necessarily enough to make them dissatisfied). We knew from several research studies that earlier concerns that implants might cause cancer were probably unfounded. And finally we knew that there were anecdotes that breast implants caused connective tissue disease, but the question had not been properly studied. Thirty years' experience, however, argued that if there were such a connection, it was certainly not common. What we had, then, was a pretty good feeling for an upper bound on the frequency and seriousness of risks.[33]

Benefits were even more difficult to assess than risks, because they are entirely subjective and unique to each woman. Most women would probably not choose implants, no matter how low the risks, either for augmentation or for reconstruction after cancer surgery. But for many women who had chosen to have implants, the matter was different. For whatever reason, they expected substantial benefit or they would not have been willing to endure an unpleasant and often expensive procedure. One woman testifying before the Weiss subcommittee said, "Having my body restored eased away much of the trauma of breast cancer."[34] Many women who had implants for augmentation felt no less strongly. One woman told *Redbook* magazine, "I'm thrilled that I did it. I used to feel bottom-heavy, although I wasn't overweight. Now I'm in proportion for the first time ever."[35]

But Kessler seemed to be saying that the benefits were trivial, at least when implants were used for cosmetic purposes, and that therefore the FDA would tolerate almost no risks. He was willing to cut a little slack for women who chose implants after cancer surgery, but only if they agreed to the inconvenience and lack of privacy entailed in being a part of a research study. But as for augmentation, Kessler said, "It makes little sense for the FDA to consider breast augmentation of equivalent importance with an accepted component of cancer therapy."[36] (This last, of course, was a stretch, in that the implants are not, strictly speaking, a part of the therapy. A mastectomy can be performed without reconstruction, and usually is.) In waving aside the benefits of breast implants for most women who had them, Kessler appeared to be introducing an impossibly high standard for the devices: since there were no benefits, there should be no risks.

At the time of the ban, the political context in which the FDA's action occurred was shifting markedly. The role of regulation in American life has grown increasingly contentious over the last decade or so, particularly since the Republican sweep of Congress in 1994. Not surprisingly, the FDA and, particularly, David Kessler have been special targets of Newt Gingrich's troops. Some of the new breed take the libertarian position that people should be free to choose their own drugs and devices; those that work will stay on the market, those that don't won't (perhaps by killing off their customers). According to this swashbuckling view, the FDA deprives people of choice and interferes with the wonders of a free market.[37] There can't be many knowledgeable people who subscribe to such silliness, but still, there is a real issue here. When should individuals in a free society have the right to make choices, even dangerous ones, and when should the government protect them?

Regulatory agencies such as the FDA were established in large part to deal with the inevitable gap in information between consumers and those promoting the product being regulated. Congress passed the Food, Drug, and Cosmetic Act in 1938, in the midst of the New Deal, to monitor the safety of food and drugs. How many Americans would be capable of deciding for themselves whether a new antibiotic actually works and what its side effects will be? How many could determine the likely performance of a new artificial heart valve? And how many would be willing to take the risk of being wrong? The medical "market" regulated by the FDA is very different from, say, a market in tennis shoes or television sets, in which choices can be made pretty easily and, in any case, the human cost of a mistake is small. Kessler is right: caveat emptor should not be the watchword of the FDA. But in the case of breast implants, as Kessler admitted, the FDA didn't know much more than the consumers. No one, in fact, could do more than make seat-of-the-pants judgments based on the same 30 years' practical, clinical experience—an experience that suggested the risks were small. To be sure, the implant manufacturers had been derelict in failing to assemble the evidence required of them. However, the FDA action was ostensibly taken not to punish them, but for the avowed purpose of protecting consumers. If the information gap between consumers and the FDA had been great and the risks large, the action would have been easily justifiable, but neither of these conditions obtained. It was therefore a matter of the FDA's judgment as to whether the risks (both known and unknown) were worth taking versus the judgment of women who might want implants. The tension was clearly between protection and choice.

Adding to this tension was the disparity between the FDA's attitude toward breast implants and the enormous range of risks that Americans are free to take quite regularly—cigarette smoking, drinking, mountain climbing, motorcycle racing, and worse. What sense does it make for a woman to be able to smoke two packs of cigarettes a day, but not be able to obtain breast implants? Kessler could counter—and probably would—that these other risks are not his business. His business is to regulate drugs and devices, and that is what he is doing. (He has taken steps to bring cigarettes under FDA purview, but the effort, while supported by President Clinton, is being hard fought by the cigarette manufacturers and members of Congress from tobacco-producing states.[38]) Nevertheless, the FDA does not exist in a vacuum, and for society as a whole, the haphazard nature of regulation is odd. Furthermore, attempting to eliminate risks nearly always introduces other risks, which may or may not be anticipated. If, for example, inspecting meat lessens the incidence of food poisoning, it also increases the price of meat. The increased cost of food for a poor family might very well reduce the family's ability to pay for medical care or housing—perhaps with more dire health consequences than occasional cases of food poisoning. More to the point, it is possible that some women may delay getting breast cancer diagnosed and treated if they cannot obtain implants for reconstruction outside a research study. Such trade-offs are rarely explicitly considered in developing regulations, yet they may be substantial. Indeed, if the risks being regulated are fairly small, the hazards of regulating them may well be higher.

Women activists seemed to be sharply divided about the breast implant ban. Some women were angry that they had been deprived of the option of having silicone breast implants. In an argument reminiscent of the abortion controversy, they claimed the issue was whether they had the right to make their own choice. They objected to the government treating them like little girls. On the March 30, 1992, Jenny Jones show, one woman, saying she had informed herself thoroughly before getting her implants, said she now worried that she would not be able to replace them if they ruptured. She went on to say, "It's not for everybody, but leave us that choice. This is our choice." Jones herself, no fan of implants, agreed that women should have the ultimate choice.[39]

In contrast, other women were convinced that breast augmentation was something that had been thrust on them by a male-dominated society obsessed with impossible notions of women's beauty. According to this view, women do not *choose* breast implants, any more than African women choose clitoridectomy or Chinese women once chose to bind their feet. They are coerced. Naomi Wolf took this argument further. In her view, part of the reason for the coercion is precisely be-

cause the procedure maims women. Said Wolf, "It is not coincidental that breast surgery is expanding at a time when female sexuality is such a threat."[40] Women who take some vari-
ant of this view are naturally disposed to accept the theory that
breast implants are dangerous.

I have no tally of how many women are on each side, but
I suspect the great majority who have opinions on the issue believe that breast implants are risky, that there is solid evidence
to this effect (some of which the manufacturers have with-
held), and that, if anything, Kessler was too slow in moving to
protect women. Some are sure he would have moved much
faster if men's health had been at risk.

In 1995 the Republican-dominated Congress initiated efforts to weaken the power of government regulation. It began
by passing legislation that would require federal regulators to
compare the costs of regulations with their benefits. On the
surface, this is a reasonable reform. The problem is that it can
become a cover for a general rollback of the philosophy that
underlies regulation—namely, that citizens need to be pro-
tected from the excesses of an unbridled market. According
to the Republicans, the federal regulatory apparatus has grown
bloated and hinders legitimate private enterprise. It needs to
be curbed for the sake of common sense and efficient government. What they are less likely to emphasize is the fact that
undermining government regulation, particularly standards
to protect the environment, is enormously appealing to big
business. The Democrats, in their typical mode these days, responded by agreeing that regulatory reform is a good idea,
but not too much of it. They maintain that the Republican
proposals will add to red tape, instead of cutting it, because
they will merely add roadblocks to the current regulations. In
the midst of this debate, Kessler is likely to emerge as an in-

creasingly popular target.[41] His strongly activist approach and the public nature of his stands on a variety of issues, including breast implants and cigarettes, make him a well-recognized symbol of government regulation. In addition, FDA rules are major obstacles to many segments of the powerful drug, device, and biotechnology industry. Although Kessler was appointed by a Republican president, he is now championed largely by Democrats, who find him much more congenial to their philosophy. It is unclear, however, whether Democratic support will be enough to protect him from the politics of regulation. If he leaves the FDA, it will almost certainly signal a much weakened agency.

Before banning breast implants, Kessler agonized about the decision publicly and, no doubt, privately. He could foresee many of the criticisms of a ban, and he was aware of the scientific shakiness of his action. What he almost certainly could not foresee, however, because of its extraordinary sweep, was the frenzy of litigation touched off by the ban.

4

THE RUSH TO COURT: LITIGATION AND MORE LITIGATION

Get your lawyers who can help you help your-selves. That's what it's all about.

—Denise Dunleavey, plaintiffs' attorney,

on "Jenny Jones,"

March 30, 1992

The FDA ban was followed by a tidal wave of litigation. In the next two years, more than 16,000 lawsuits, brought by over a thousand lawyers, on behalf of women with breast implants were filed in federal and state courts.[1] Dow Corning alone saw a surge in lawsuits from about 200 at the end of 1991 to 10,000 by the end of 1992.[2] As Jack Weinstein, the senior federal judge for the Eastern District of New York who presided over the Agent Orange class action, observed, "The speed with which the number of breast implant cases exploded on the scene is attributable in part to a well-organized plaintiffs' bar, which now has the capital, organizational skills, and advertising techniques to seek clientele."[3] A small display advertisement in the July 26, 1994, *Washington Post* exemplified the spirit: "The law firm of Chandler, Franklin, and O'Brien is pleased to announce the opening of our new Fairfax office devoted exclusively to representing women in breast implant litigation," followed by the toll-free number, 1-800-488-4LAW. For those who preferred, Kresch & Kresch could be reached at 1-800-LAW-HELP, or a Florida attorney at 1-800-RUPTURE.[4] According to Barie Carmichael, corporate vice-president of Dow Corning, computer networking among plaintiffs' attorneys made it possible to generate lawsuits with unprecedented speed. Interested lawyers could easily learn the status of relevant lawsuits throughout the country and modify the wording of promising ones for their own use. By the time of the class settlement, Dow Corning claimed to be the target of 30,000 lawsuits, many of which were evidently clones, since they contained the same typographical errors.[5] Even as all but two of the manufacturers went out of the implant business, the number of lawyers belonging to Public Citizen's breast implant clearinghouse increased from 4 in 1990 to 179 in 1992,[6] and the Breast Implant Committee of the Association of Trial Lawyers of America (an organization of plaintiffs' attorneys) grew from 20 to 160 in just the six months leading up to the ban.[7]

The flood of breast implant lawsuits was simply one more manifestation of Americans' fervor for suing one another (or threatening to). As Harvard law professor Mary Ann Glendon said in her book, *A Nation under Lawyers,* "While some lawyers were touting litigation as a quick fix for social ills, others were teaching that for nearly every injury suffered by a private individual there is someone with deep pockets, the government or a large corporation, who can be sued and made to pay."[8] The sheer size of the court system buttresses her point. At the end of the 1980s, about 18 million civil lawsuits were filed annually in state and federal courts[9]—one lawsuit for every ten adults in the United States. Nearly 2 million of these were tort cases[10]—that is, they involved seeking monetary damages for product liability, medical malpractice, or other personal injury. Although the rate of increase in tort cases has been modest over the last decade or so,[11] that does not tell the whole story. About three-quarters of tort claims are settled before a lawsuit is filed, and there is evidence that the number of these settlements is rising rapidly. Even those that are filed are usually settled before trial; only about 3 percent of personal injury claims ever come before a jury.[12] Nevertheless, there are changes in the pattern of tort cases that justify concerns about a litigation explosion. First, mass personal injury litigation—thousands of lawsuits involving the same product or injury, such as the breast implant litigation—has burgeoned, particularly since 1980.[13] And second, the size of jury awards has grown rapidly. In particular, punitive damages against manufacturers, while still rare, have grown enormously.[14] Thus, despite the fact that the absolute number of lawsuits has not increased dramatically, the total costs of the tort system increased from $46.6 billion to $132.2 billion in the decade 1980 to 1990 (accounting for about 2.3 percent of the gross domestic product at the end of the decade).[15] Solid data, however, are hard to come by, and these figures must be taken as only approximate. The direction, however, is clear.

The number of lawyers has also increased. Whereas there were 542,205 lawyers in the United States in 1980, at the end of the decade there were 805,872. We now have about 900,000 lawyers in the country.[16] Only a minority are trial lawyers, although no one seems to know for sure what that percentage is and how fast it is growing. One way to look at the increasing numbers of lawyers is that they are merely keeping pace with the demand. But it is also plausible that lawyers to a great extent *create* their demand. Certainly, like doctors, they have a good deal of latitude to generate their own business. If a lawyer says you need him or her, it's difficult to argue, just as it may be risky to argue with your doctor. In any case, lawyers no longer simply wait for clients. Instead, they actively seek them out. Soliciting clients was once universally condemned by the bar, but it is now fairly standard practice. Lawyers even appeal for clients on television. In one series of ads, for example, a Massachusetts medical malpractice lawyer, looking lugubriously at the camera, urges sympathetically, "Don't go it alone. Let us help you get the help you need." Advertisements also appear in newspapers and magazines, often with 800 numbers containing the letters *LAW*.

Glendon believes that excessive litigation is an unforeseen fallout of the 1960s. In that decade, according to her thesis, we began to turn to the courts to rectify nearly all social ills and injustices. This has become an expensive habit, she argues, which is accompanied by atrophy of the more traditional, but slower methods of effecting change—including the political process. People sue one another, instead of voting. As lawsuits have proliferated since the 1960s, the character of the legal profession has itself changed. No longer does it emphasize negotiation and conciliation, or measure success by whether litigation can be avoided. Now it emphasizes rights and combat, and success is measured by how big you win in court. Even within the staid academic community, the legal hero is no longer the corporate lawyer, but the trial lawyer, and winning a weak case is even more celebrated than winning a strong one. Harvard is proud of Alan Dershowitz.

Whatever the strength of Glendon's thesis, there are also more prosaic reasons for Americans to turn to the law when they are ill or hurt. As the advanced nation most committed to an unbridled free market, this country can be a harsh place.

Big business is powerful and often ruthless, and the safety net for those who suffer harms of whatever kind is notoriously threadbare. In particularly, medical care is expensive and by no means assured for everyone who needs it. Thus, people who are injured or sick have every interest in blaming the problem on someone else and trying to collect damages. A successful lawsuit may be the only way to provide for medical expenses and lost income (often called "economic" damages). Sometimes there are also damages for emotional harm, and these may be at least as large as the economic damages. Finally, punitive damages are awarded in some cases. Although punitive damages are rare, they receive a great deal more publicity than their frequency warrants, because they may be huge. For example, in one breast implant case, the plaintiff was awarded $5 million in economic and emotional damages, and $20 million in punitive damages.[17] The size of punitive damages reflects their purpose; they are designed to punish or deter the defendant. They are therefore based on the defendant's wealth and must be big enough to be felt. In one breast implant case, the jury was instructed that the net worth of the defendant, Dow Corning, was over $948 million, a figure the jury was to keep in mind when deciding on punitive damages.[18] Although the great majority of product liability cases are settled out of court, there are enough multimillion-dollar jury verdicts to remind manufacturers that settling is usually better. Losing just one case can generate multiple similar cases and set the minimum going rate for compensation. The threat of punitive damages is an added wild card.

American law has a number of unusual, even unique, features that contribute to the large and growing number of lawsuits. First, we alone use the contingency fee as the customary method of payment of plaintiffs' attorneys in personal injury cases. By this method the attorney is paid a percentage of the plaintiff's award. If the plaintiff loses, the attorney may get nothing. But if the plaintiff wins, the usual contingency fee is a third of the award, plus expenses.[19] Other countries do not use contingency fees, and Great Britain does not permit them.[20] In this country, it is argued, they are necessary because many plaintiffs could not afford to sue without this arrangement, given the high fees of lawyers. The problem is that the contingency-fee system makes a lottery of the process and entices plaintiffs and lawyers to play the game. It provides an incentive for lawyers to sue frequently, with scant consideration of the merits of the case. Even though they expect to lose most cases, every now and then they will win a large verdict that can subsidize the losses. The high costs of defending against multiple lawsuits generated by the contingency system are incentives for defendants to settle even weak cases out of court. On the other hand, plaintiffs' attorneys may be quick to settle even strong cases, rather than go through the rigors of a trial. In either case, justice is not well served.

Another unusual feature of the American tort system is the use of juries.[21] Most other countries reserve juries for criminal cases, but we also permit jury trials for tort cases, as well as other civil cases in which monetary damages are sought. The presence of juries increases the lottery aspects of the tort system. Skillful plaintiffs' attorneys may select only the most appealing clients, and focus their efforts primarily on mobilizing the sympathy of the jury. Sometimes, they draw on consultants in jury selection to choose a jury most likely to be sympathetic to a particular client. (Defense attorneys, for their part, try to select unsympathetic jurors.) The resultant verdict may have little to do with the merits of the case, and everything to do with theater. If things go well, a sympathetic jury may award large damages for emotional distress, as well as economic damages. The outcome is a gamble for high stakes. An attorney may have to file a lot of lawsuits to ensure a big win from time to time. The capriciousness of this system—the disconnection between the merits of the case and the verdict—ought to be sobering to those who care about justice, but it certainly is good business for the plaintiffs' bar.

A RELATIVELY NEW and controversial movement in tort law is the use of class actions and multidistrict consolidations to deal with multiple lawsuits involving the same kind of product or injury or the same defendants. Such mass tort litigation is becoming increasingly common, in part because large numbers of people are more likely to be exposed to the same injurious agent or event. According to a report by the Institute for Civil Justice, a research arm of RAND, "The 1980's marked the era of mass personal injury litigation. Hundreds of thousands of people sued scores of corporations for losses due to injuries or diseases that they attributed to catastrophic events, pharmaceutical products, medical devices, or toxic substances."[22] The era was presaged in 1973, when the first successful product liability litigation against asbestos manufacturers was decided. Ultimately, well over 200,000 lawsuits were filed against multiple manufacturers of asbestos. Other mass tort litigation soon followed. Beginning in the 1970s and continuing into the 1990s, over a thousand lawsuits were filed against Eli Lilly, Abbott Laboratories, and other drug companies on behalf of women who developed vaginal carcinoma because their mothers took the drug diethylstilbestrol (DES) to prevent miscarriage.[23] Starting about the same time and continuing into the mid-1980s, 1,800 lawsuits were initiated against Merrell Dow Pharmaceuticals claiming that the drug Bendectin, given to prevent morning sickness during pregnancy, had caused birth defects.[24] Nearly 200,000 women sued A. H. Robins alleging damage from the Dalkon Shield intrauterine contraceptive device[25]; 250,000 sued the makers of Agent Orange (dioxin)[26]; 50,000 sued Pfizer, Inc., the makers of the defective Bjork-Shiley artificial heart valve[27]; and so on. By the 1980s, mass tort cases were commonplace. The next mass litigation to rival the breast implant case may be based on alleged damage from lead paint. A story in the August 14, 1995, *New York Times* described the liability explosion facing New York City from nearly a thousand claims filed on behalf of children exposed to lead paint in city-owned buildings. The report predicted that resolving the cases already filed could cost the city as much as $500 million.[28] These cases will surely be followed by others. It is important to recognize that the size and outcome of mass tort litigation may have very little to do with the actual risk of the product. Among the mass litigation cases I have mentioned, the products present widely varying degrees of risk. Some, such as DES, are clearly dangerous; others, such as asbestos, are dangerous only under certain circumstances; and others, such as Bendectin, have been well studied and shown to be safe.

When large numbers of people claim to be injured by the same product, individual lawsuits can be an extremely inefficient and capricious way to deal with the claims. Plaintiffs have to race one another to court to try to collect damages and hope they get there before the defendants run out of money. Verdicts vary greatly and seemingly arbitrarily. As an example, the asbestos mass litigation is generally agreed to have been a disaster. The courts were flooded, with chaotic and uneven results. Many of the cases are still unsettled. In 1982, Johns-Manville, a major manufacturer of asbestos, filed for Chapter 11 bankruptcy protection. This was the company's only option for dealing with both federal and state cases at the same time. Chapter 11 bankruptcy entails the financial reorganization of a company, not its liquidation. As a part of the reorganization, all creditors' claims are considered together in a single court—the bankruptcy court. Asbestos suits against Johns-Manville Corporation must now be resolved by a claims facility, the Manville Personal Injury Settlement Trust. The damages will be paid only at greatly reduced rates, if at all. Eventually 17 other companies involved in the manufacture or use of asbestos also filed for bankruptcy protection. Similarly, A. H. Robins, the manufacturer of the Dalkon Shield, filed for bankruptcy protection, leaving the claims of many women unsettled. They will be resolved by the Dalkon Shield Claimants' Trust Facility.[29] There was very little equity among the plaintiffs in these cases. Early claimants tended to fare better than late ones. The large punitive damages early plaintiffs received simply increased the likelihood that the companies went bankrupt before those injured last could file their claims.

The filing of class actions—lawsuits in which the plaintiffs are alleged to represent a large number of similarly affected people—is one way to deal with the inequities and inefficiencies of mass torts. Class actions have long been used for civil cases involving injunctions—such as those dealing with school segregation and job discrimination. What is new since the 1970s is the use of class actions in tort cases. Until the 1970s, the general rule was one lawyer, one client.[30] But with the explosion in mass tort litigation, it has become increasingly common for plaintiffs' attorneys to file class actions. A class needs to be certified by a federal judge, who must be satisfied that class-action treatment is the best method for reaching a fair and efficient resolution of the problem. The judge not only certifies the class, but also chooses the class representative, in whose name the lawsuit is filed on behalf of the other members of the class. The judge also selects the lead attorneys for the class and approves their fees.[31] Pooling cases raises the stakes enough to warrant hiring experts and conducting an exhaustive pretrial investigation. The plaintiffs' lawyers in essence become investors in the process.

Although attorneys' fees for a class action tend to be a smaller percentage than the standard one-third contingency fee, they are nevertheless quite large because of the number of plaintiffs. Filing a class action can therefore be a very lucrative proposition, and there is great competition to be chosen to represent the class. Recall that the breast implant settlement explicitly set aside a billion dollars for the lawyers.[32] For this reason, class actions are now filed on behalf of all sorts of dubious groups. Sometimes multiple class actions are filed against the same manufacturer. For example, there have already been 46 class actions filed against Wyeth-Ayerst, the manufacturer of Norplant.[33] Here again, there is a lottery aspect to the practice. Most class actions are not certified, but all it takes is one to make an attorney's career. A class action may be settled out of court either before or after the class is certified. When the attorneys for both sides agree on the settlement after a class has been certified, the judge decides whether it is fundamentally fair, then notifies the members of the class of a formal hearing in which they can present arguments for and against the settlement. The judge then either approves or disapproves the settlement.[34]

Often mass tort litigation involves plaintiffs from multiple federal districts. In this case, it is necessary to consolidate the cases within the jurisdiction of one federal court. In 1968, Congress created the Judicial Panel on Multidistrict Litigation. This group of judges is authorized to transfer civil actions involving common questions of fact from multiple districts to one. The purpose is to consolidate pretrial discovery—that is, to conduct out-of-court questioning of parties and witnesses. The defendants and their witnesses need present their documents and answers to plaintiffs' inquiries only once. The cases may then be completed in their original districts, or, as in the breast implant class action, settled together. States may also consolidate mass tort litigation within one state court. Because mass tort litigation is still a relatively new field, the procedures are fairly flexible or confused, depending on your point of view. There is no question that the phenomenon involves a good deal of legal pioneering.[35]

In early 1992, Stanley Chesley, the Cincinnati lawyer who pioneered class actions in tort cases, sought to have the breast implant cases treated as a class under his sole control. Chesley's action provoked outrage from his colleagues, who charged that his real interest was the large fee that would accrue to him if he were named to manage the settlement. In 1983, Chesley had managed to get the 250,000 Vietnam veterans who claimed to be injured by Agent Orange certified as a class. The case was ultimately settled for $180 million (Chesley received over $525,000 for his efforts). Since then, he has made a specialty of class-action settlements. Other plaintiffs' attorneys tend to be highly critical of him, ostensibly because he is too quick to settle for too little. (Of course, they also lose clients to him.) Initially Chesley got Judge Carl Rubin, an Ohio federal judge, to certify the implant recipients as a class. When other plaintiffs' attorneys complained to the Judicial Panel on Multidistrict Litigation, the panel transferred all federal cases to Alabama federal judge Sam C. Pointer, an expert in complex litigation. He appointed a 17-member plaintiffs steering committee, headed by Chesley and Atlanta trial attorney Ralph Knowles, to work out a settlement with the manufacturers.

The choice was diplomatic. Just as Chesley was a known champion of class actions, so Knowles had been a leader of the Breast Implant Litigation Group of the Association of Trial Lawyers of America, a group not enamored of class actions.[36]

Two years later, on April 1, 1994, a proposed settlement of the class action was finally approved by both sides.[37] The terms, revised over the next few weeks, were remarkably generous and broad. They provided for $4.25 billion to be set aside for all women who had received breast implants of any type before June 1, 1993—and their lawyers. Every effort was made to help women make claims. The court compiled an enormous list of all women thought to have breast implants, based on multiple sources of information. Each woman was mailed a comprehensive but readable description of the terms of the settlement, a registration form, a claim form, and a form to opt out of the settlement if she wished. Conditions that would be compensated were listed, along with the criteria for diagnosis. A very simple question-and-answer booklet was also included, and a toll-free number for any additional questions.

According to the settlement, all women with breast implants were entitled to compensation if they had, or within the next 30 years developed, any of 10 connective tissue diseases or symptoms suggestive of such diseases, provided the symptoms began or worsened after the implants were placed. Of the $4.25 billion contributed by the manufacturers, $1.2 billion was set aside for women claiming to have already developed implant-related illnesses. By June 1, 1995, 248,500 women claimed to have such illnesses. The amount of compensation they were entitled to was determined by the type of disorder, its severity, and the woman's age at onset. A chart or "grid" sent to all women with breast implants showed the exact amounts to be paid. For example, according to the grid, a woman under age thirty-six with severe scleroderma would receive $1.4 million; a woman over age fifty-six with mild Sjögren's syndrome (dryness of the eyes and salivary glands) would receive $140,000. Claimants did not need to show that the implants were related to the illness. In addition, women who were not ill could receive lesser amounts for emotional distress. They would also be reimbursed for all uninsured medical costs related to breast implants, including evaluations, treatment of implant rupture, and elective removal of implants. Husbands and other "significant others," who presumably suffered emotionally from the situation, and children born before April 1, 1994, were also entitled to make claims. Children, for example, could claim compensation for injuries caused by their mothers' implants (a particularly mysterious provision, since no such condition has ever been demonstrated).

Women claiming current illness were required to submit substantiating medical records. If these were not sufficient to place the woman in the appropriate category on the grid, the woman's doctor was to send the diagnosis, along with copies of relevant records. Beyond this, there would be no attempt to verify the woman's condition. A doctor's diagnosis or the medical records would be challenged only if they failed to meet the eligibility requirements. Many of the eligibility requirements can be objectively measured, such as swollen joints or abnormal substances in the blood. But some cannot, such as fatigue or muscle aches. Indeed, it would have been possible to qualify for compensation without any objective manifestations of illness whatsoever. For example, a woman could claim joint and muscle aches, disturbed sleep, fatigue, and burning pain in the chest, none of which can be objectively verified by her doctor or anyone else, and collect up to $700,000.[38]

All this assumed that the settlement held together. There were, however, two hitches that made that unlikely from the beginning. First, any of the defendants could back out of the class-action settlement if they believed its purpose was being defeated by too many women opting out and pursuing large individual settlements or jury awards. And second, if too many women made claims under the class settlement, the amount of compensation for each woman would have to be decreased. According to the settlement terms, if the grid were revised women would then be given another opportunity to opt out. Because of these conditions, as well as the generous terms and loose requirements for verification, the class settlement began to unravel almost as soon as it was put together.[39] More about that later.

IN THE FRENZY of litigation that followed the FDA ban, it did not take long for some plaintiffs' attorneys to realize that they could very easily extend their reach to other silicone-containing medical devices. One target is penile implants. Once again the class action is a favored method of enterprising lawyers. In 1994 Dan Bolton, of breast implant fame, filed a class-action lawsuit in the U.S. District Court in San Francisco on behalf of three Northern California men with penile implants and roughly 300,000 others. He claimed that the devices, in addition to causing local complications, could damage the body's immune system.[40] Penile implants are made by American Medical Systems, a subsidiary of Pfizer. Like breast implants, they came under FDA purview in 1976 and were grandfathered. Bolton is quoted as saying, "In many ways this case is very similar to the court battles waged against the manufacturers of breast implants," and he ought to know.[41] Other attorneys also filed class actions against American Medical Systems, one of which asked for $50,000 per class member.

Perhaps the most interesting fallout of breast implant lit-igation is the new wariness about Norplant, the implantable contraceptive introduced in 1991. Norplant is placed under the skin of the arm in six very small, silicone-coated rods. Its effects last for five years. Because users need not think about it, Norplant, approved by the FDA in 1990, is probably the most reliable contraceptive on the market, particularly for teenagers.[42] However, it has suddenly become a target for product liability suits similar to those against breast implant manufacturers. The number of lawsuits against Wyeth-Ayerst, the manufacturer of Norplant, and the parent company, American Home Products, rose from 20 in the first three years that Norplant was on the market to 180 in 1994. In addition, as already mentioned, nearly 50 class-action suits have been filed. Dr. Elizabeth Connell, professor of gynecology and ob-stetrics at Emory University and the chair of the 1992 FDA panel on breast implants, told the *New York Times* that the par-allels between the breast implant and Norplant controversies are striking. In both cases, lawyers have been actively recruit-ing women to sue manufacturers, and some medical experts involved in the suits own laboratories that purport to test for silicone-related illnesses—even though such tests are of un-proven value. The first National Norplant Litigation Confer-ence, to instruct lawyers and doctors on how to participate in Norplant litigation, was held in Houston in June 1995. Some of the lawyers who organized it are also heavily involved in breast implant litigation. The illnesses attributed to Norplant are similar to those said to be caused by breast implants, in-cluding autoimmune and connective-tissue-like disorders and neurologic problems. There is no medical evidence to impli-cate Norplant in these disorders, but the fears are real enough. Norplant use has plummeted from 800 implants a day to 60.[43] The untoward consequences of trying to eliminate all theoretical risks are easily seen in this case. Would any silicone-associated risks outweigh the many risks and costs of unwanted pregnancies in women who are frightened away from Norplant and unable to use another contraceptive?

More important than the expansion of litigation to other silicone-containing products is the indirect threat to all medical devices—whether they contain silicone or not. This threat arises from a peculiar feature of our product liability laws. According to the law, plaintiffs can make claims against any party involved in the manufacture of an allegedly harmful product, even if the involvement is remote.[44] This means that suppliers of raw materials can be sued, even if they have nothing to do with the design and manufacture of the product. Since the sale of raw materials for medical devices (called biomaterials) is a small part of the business of most big suppliers, some of them have calculated that their revenues from this stream would quickly be dwarfed by the legal liabilities. For example, DuPont once supplied Teflon to a small company, called Vitek, that used it to manufacture jaw implants. Several years ago, when there were problems with the implants, Vitek declared bankruptcy. The aggrieved patients then sued DuPont instead. Although the courts have ruled fairly consistently in favor of DuPont, the company estimates it spent about $8 million a year over five years defending itself against the suits. This amounted to far more than the return on the five cents' worth of Teflon in each implant.[45]

Ostensibly because of the legal risks, three large suppliers of biomaterials have pulled back from the market. Dow Corning, a supplier as well as a manufacturer, has drastically scaled back sales of silicone to other manufacturers of medical devices and may stop selling it altogether. The embargo will probably affect a wide variety of silicone-containing de-

vices, ranging from useful to vital. Among them are cardiac
pacemaker wires, artificial joints, mechanical heart valves, in-
traocular lenses (used after cataract surgery), implantable ar-
teriovenous shunts for people on chronic dialysis, and shunts
for people with hydrocephalus (a potentially lethal condition
in which fluid accumulates in the brain). Dow Chemical Company has stopped supplying a material used in pacemaker
components. DuPont announced in 1993 that it would sever
connections with the permanent medical implant industry in
1994. It would no longer supply medical manufacturers with
Dacron polyester (used in vascular grafts), Teflon, or a number of other biomaterials. In DuPont's calculus, what had happened with silicone could happen with any other constituent
of medical devices.[46]

Under these conditions, a large number of very important
medical products may become scarce or even unavailable. At
the least, they will become more expensive. In May 1994, Senator Joseph Lieberman (D-Conn.), then chairman of the Governmental Affairs Subcommittee on Regulation and Government Information, held hearings on the impact of product
liability suits on the availability of medical devices. Among
those who testified was the father of a boy with hydrocephalus.
The boy, like many other people with hydrocephalus, is able
to live a normal life because the fluid in his brain is shunted
to his abdominal cavity by a silicone tube. Without the shunt,
he would die. But the shunt needs to be replaced periodically
as the boy grows. It can also break, requiring immediate replacement. The father testified that he lives in fear that shunts
for hydrocephalus may become unavailable.[47]

Also testifying at the Lieberman hearings was Eleanor
Gackstatter, president of Meadox Medicals, a manufacturer of
vascular grafts and other devices. She said that she had tried

to contact 15 alternative suppliers of polyester yarn after DuPont announced it would no longer supply Dacron to her company. None of them, even foreign suppliers, would deal with American manufacturers because of the liability risks. Many manufacturers have a two- or three-year supply of biomaterials on hand, but when that is depleted, there may be a serious shortage. Senator Lieberman, arguing for reform of the product liability system, said, "This is a public health time bomb, and the lives of real people are going to be lost if it explodes."[48]

Norplant and penile implants are important to those who use them, of course, but an argument can be made that, as elective devices, no great damage is being done by the threat to their availability. It is far harder to accept the wholesale threat to vital medical devices, regardless of whether they contain silicone. How this tale will unfold as scarcity develops is impossible to predict. Some critics believe that the suppliers are withholding biomaterials only for political reasons. According to this view, suppliers are cynically attempting to create a backlash against the product liability system.[49] On the other hand, the facts of the matter are clear; suppliers of biomaterials *can* be held liable for products they have not designed, manufactured, or sold. And if, for this reason, the suppliers continue to refuse biomaterials to American manufacturers of medical devices, some of the manufacturers may find it necessary to relocate abroad.

The destructive effects of a runaway tort system are not what juries are thinking about when they award large damages to plaintiffs. They are thinking about the plaintiff's case. People who have been injured, by bad luck or careless behavior, as well as by a defective product, look for some way to get help. Since there is no reliable social system in the United States for caring for the sick or injured, it is left to the tort system. Some plaintiffs are vastly rewarded; most are not. The connection between the verdict and the merits of the case is often tenuous. Compassionate people may welcome large verdicts for plaintiffs (and as jurors, they are happy to provide them). Some believe that even if the injury was not caused by the defendant, it could have been and, besides, someone should compensate the victim. But this is a very haphazard and uneconomical way to provide assistance. As a way to deter businesses from marketing dangerous products, the system also fails. To be sure, businesses grow more skittish, but the issue for them becomes not whether a product is actually safe, but whether the company will be vulnerable. They may shy away from important innovations just to minimize their liability. Finally, as a way to redistribute wealth, the system fails utterly. Since someone must pay for the jury awards, the costs are merely passed along to ordinary consumers. For example, the breast implant manufacturers will surely try to recoup their losses by increasing the prices of their other consumer goods. (Such price increases are sometimes called a "tort tax.")

Tort reform, like regulatory reform, has been a recurrent theme in Washington, but never more than now in the ultra-conservative Republican Congress. Various reform measures have been proposed. These include limitations on the size of punitive and emotional damages, as well as restrictions on contingency fees and more stringent standards for the admissibility of scientific evidence in court. In addition, there has been increasing attention to the problems of remote parties, such as suppliers of biomaterials, drawn into product liability suits. Product liability suits pit trial lawyers against big business. Each side has its champions. Republicans and conservatives tend to support big business. They are therefore eager to reform the tort system to limit contingency fees and punitive damages. Democrats and liberals, on the other hand, see themselves as championing the average citizen, and tend to support the plaintiffs' lawyers. They believe that retaining the present tort system, with all its incentives to sue, gives everyone a day in court and is necessary to protect consumers from unscrupulous business practices.[50]

Although the view of the tort system tends to split along party lines, with Democrats being more willing to tolerate the abuses of the system and Republicans likely to seize on them as an excuse to indulge big business, attitudes are no longer as predictable as they once were. Even so thoroughgoing a liberal as former senator George McGovern said, in 1994, "America is in the midst of a new Civil War, a war that threatens to undercut the civil basis of our society. It is a war of lawsuits. . . . We need more hard information on campaign contributions and lobbying by the trial lawyers. I have no hesitance in asserting that this lobby is one of the most potent and selfish bands in Washington."[51] Indeed, plaintiffs' attorneys have emerged as one of the largest single groups of contributors for political office anywhere in the United States, particularly at the state level. According to the American Tort Reform Association, a nonprofit group of about 400 organizations interested in tort reform, from 1990 to 1994 plaintiffs' attorneys contributed more for state and local candidates in just three states (Alabama, Texas, and California) than either the Republican or Democratic National Committees did in all 50 states. In Texas alone, they are said to have contributed $8.8 million to candidates for state office, including candidates for the Texas Supreme Court.[52] I will revisit Texas later.

The rush to court following the FDA ban on breast implants has had, as we have seen, immense effects on commerce and the law, as well as on hundreds of thousands of women with breast implants. But what is the truth about breast implants? Are all the anguish, expense, and shifts in fortune justified? To answer these questions, we need to turn to science, which was conspicuous by its absence as the breast implant story developed.

5

SCIENTIFIC EVIDENCE: WHAT IT IS AND WHERE IT COMES FROM

We found no association between breast implants and the connective tissue diseases and other disorders we studied.

—Mayo Clinic researcher Dr. Sherine Gabriel,
June 16, 1994

Whether silicone-gel-filled breast implants cause connective tissue disease is not ultimately a matter of opinion or legal argument; it is a matter of biological fact. Either they cause connective tissue disease (alone or in conjunction with other factors) or they don't. Plaintiffs' attorneys, consumer advocates, implant manufacturers, and scientists can debate the point as loudly and insistently as they like, but the noise of the debate should not be allowed to obscure the basic truth that the question has an answer and the answer lies in nature. The only way to learn whether breast implants cause connective tissue disease is by scientific studies.

Science plays a hugely important role in our daily lives, and not just because we are dependent on its technological fruits. In addition, we base many of our habits and activities on the results of research studies, as interpreted for us by the media. Medical research, in particular, increasingly informs our lives. We are subject to an almost incessant barrage of warnings and recommendations based on new medical information. Yet, despite the practical importance of science in our lives, most Americans find the nature of scientific research a complete mystery. To many of them, the conclusion is all that matters. It's as though Americans said to medical researchers, "Tell us what we should and shouldn't eat, which vitamins to take, and how much to exercise, and don't bother us with how you found the answers or how sure you are." But in science, the conclusions cannot be separated from the process of reaching them. We must know something about the way scientists work before we can begin to make sense of medical news.

Without some knowledge of the scientific process, people tend to be whipsawed by speculation, pseudo-science, and preliminary hints, many of which are contradictory. Furthermore, not knowing the broad contours of the process feeds the false belief that medical research is somehow too complex to be understood by nonscientists. This may be true of the details of any given study, but it is not true of the broad outlines. The general approach is easy to understand, because it is largely a matter of common sense. If nonscientists had a better feeling for the approach, they could gauge the probable strength of many scientific claims while knowing very little of the technical details on which they are based. Because I believe so strongly that most nonscientists can understand much more than they think they can about medical research, I will discuss some of the general principles of the scientific approach, before illustrating them (often in absentia) in the breast implant case.

Perhaps the most important hallmark of science is its utter reliance on evidence. Furthermore, the evidence must be objectively verifiable. This reliance on concrete evidence distinguishes science from all other human endeavors. To some, the reliance is unpalatable. It renders science somehow dry and a little inhuman. (Recall that in popular culture scientists are usually "nerds.") Certainly, science can seem less rich than other aspects of life, such as religion or literature, which draw on many more facets of human nature. But to many scientists who find pleasure in the search for nature's secrets, the view that science is dry is a caricature. To them, evidence anchors them to reality, which is what most fascinates them. Whether reliance on physical evidence diminishes or enhances the appeal of science is arguable. What is not arguable is that we cannot reach scientific conclusions without evidence. Medical conclusions are no different from other scientific matters, because the body is a part of nature. The effect of breast implants on women's health is no less a scientific matter than the trajectory of a lunar space shot or the impact of aerosolized sprays on the ozone layer.

How do medical researchers find the evidence on which their conclusions are based? The approach is quite uniform. First, they need to formulate the question they want to answer and design a study that is capable of answering it. The question is usually framed as a hypothesis. "Women with breast implants are more likely to develop connective tissue disease than other women" is a hypothesis.[1] (For technical reasons, it is usually framed in the negative—that is, "women with implants are *no* more likely to. . . ." This is termed the "null hypothesis," and the researcher tries to prove it wrong.) Although this first step in approaching a scientific question seems obvious and simple, mistakes are often made here. If, for example, researchers want to know whether breast implants increase the risk of connective tissue disease, they need to choose some suitable evidence of connective tissue disease and determine whether it is more common in women with implants than in women without implants. It would not be adequate to study whether women with implants are fatigued because fatigue is not specifically enough related to connective tissue disease and its presence or absence would not directly address the question. There must be a close fit between the question posed and what is being observed in the study.

After the study is designed, researchers must collect data. Collecting data means measuring or counting something. This is the notion that many nonscientists are least comfortable with, because it "reduces everything to numbers." "Everything" can't be reduced to numbers, of course, but some things can and some things must be. To reach a conclusion about the physical world (and our bodies are a part of that world), we need numbers because they are often the only way that evidence can be expressed. In a study of breast implants and connective tissue disease, for example, something must be measured or counted—the body temperature, the number of women who have joint pains, or the number of white blood cells (the cells involved in immune reactions). What is enumerated depends on the study design. When the data are assembled, they must be analyzed appropriately. Often the analysis consists of comparing one set of data with another set to lead to a logical conclusion. For example, the number of white blood cells in women with implants might be compared with the number in women without implants.

The final step in a research study, after the data are analyzed, is to draw the proper conclusions. Just as the first stage of the study (formulating the question and designing the study) is more difficult than it may at first seem, so is the last stage. Interpreting a study is perilous because of the strong temptation to reach conclusions that are more encompassing than the evidence will support. For example, if a study showed that rats injected with silicone developed cancer, it would be inaccurate to conclude that breast implants cause cancer in women. The study did not deal with women and it did not deal with implants but with liquid silicone. Similarly, if women with breast implants were found to have more white cells in their blood, it would be inaccurate to conclude that breast implants cause autoimmune disease. The study did not deal with autoimmune disease. In both of these hypothetical cases, the conclusions would go far beyond the evidence. Mistakes in drawing conclusions are particularly likely when a researcher has strong preconceptions about the question he or she is studying. The conclusions of a research study must be limited to those—and only those—that follow logically and necessarily from the data.

In science, the requirement for verifiable evidence must be met, no matter who the researchers are or what their credentials. Not even Nobel laureates are permitted to base a scientific conclusion on an educated guess. (They can, of course, make guesses or hypothesize, but those guesses will not be accepted as evidence unless they are put to the test.) These stringent standards serve a purpose. In science as in all walks of life, it's not easy to know when you have leapt to an unjustified conclusion or simply made a mistake. Sometimes very successful scientists, perhaps even more so than novices, come to believe they are more or less infallible. A distinguished senior scientist once insisted to me, when I was discussing with him the need for more data in a paper he had submitted to the *New England Journal of Medicine,* that he didn't need more data. He was, he reminded me, the discoverer of the disease that was the subject of the paper and he knew his conclusions were correct. Although he was indeed the discoverer of the disease, his eminence and expertise did not exempt him from having to produce the data required to support his conclusions. Strict adherence to scientific procedures—in particular, the requirement for evidence—saves such people (and us) from themselves.

Once a research study is completed, is that it? Do the researchers simply announce their conclusions to the media? Unfortunately, that happens from time to time, but it shouldn't. The usual procedure is for researchers to write up their study in a standardized way and submit it to a scientific journal. Research reports are divided into sections dealing with the methods, results, and conclusions. Before a research paper is published, other scientists usually evaluate the study and its conclusions. This is termed "peer review," and it is a cornerstone of scientific research. The reason peer review is so important is that even the most honest researchers cannot be expected to judge their own work dispassionately. They are likely to be enthusiastic about their ideas and, almost by definition, not aware of flaws in the design of their study and interpretation of their data. The process of interpreting data is seldom clear-cut, and it is easy to be unaware that the data are inadequate to support the conclusions. Without the discipline of organizing and presenting their evidence, and without the criticism and revisions stimulated by the peer-review process, researchers may unconsciously misrepresent their work or exaggerate its importance.

Evaluating medical research is no easy matter. At the *New England Journal of Medicine,* we have seven full-time physician editors, six part-time physician specialists, three statistical consultants, and one consultant in molecular medicine to do it, and we call on thousands of outside peer reviewers who are experts in the subjects under study.[2] Even with all this expertise, we are often not confident of the validity of a study and we sometimes make mistakes in judgment that are not corrected until later. Because of the difficulty of evaluating medical research, one should be extremely skeptical of research findings that are announced directly to the media, without peer review. The 1989 press conference of Stanley Pons and Martin Fleischmann, two chemists at the University of Utah who claimed that they had attained cold fusion, is an example of the hazards of short-circuiting the peer-review process.[3] They went directly to the media to announce that they had initiated a nuclear reaction at room temperature. According to the laws of physics, enormously high temperatures are necessary for such a reaction, yet Pons and Fleischmann were not fazed by the improbability of what they had purportedly accomplished. Neither was the University of Utah, which parlayed the spectacular announcement into a $5 million grant from the state legislature to continue the work. Later, of course, the claim could not be supported. Many other such instances could be cited in which scientists promulgate confusion or error by making claims before submitting their data to expert critical review by their professional peers.

In addition to the reliance on objective evidence collected in properly designed studies, science is also characterized by its tentativeness. This may seem counterintuitive to nonscientists who are accustomed to thinking of science as cut-and-dried. But in fact, good scientists rarely reach absolute conclusions. Particularly in medical research, certainty is extremely hard to come by. Instead, medical researchers almost always speak in terms of probabilities. When they do a study comparing two antibiotics to treat pneumonia, for example, they will couch their findings in terms of the probability that one is better than the other. When they look at the link between cholesterol and heart disease, they frame their results in terms of risks, not certainties. Very few studies are by themselves definitive. In general we should not embrace the conclusions of a research study until it has been confirmed by other, independent studies. Even then, the studies taken together merely add to the probability that the conclusion is correct, without proving it absolutely. Of course, every aspect of life involves considering probabilities. When we drive to work, for example, we intuitively gauge the probability that an oncoming car will miss us.[4] But scientific research is different in that probability and uncertainty are explicitly considered, measured, and expressed as part of the study. We can rarely absolutely prove a hypothesis, although we can gather enough evidence from enough different studies to make the hypothesis so probable that we can say it is true for all practical purposes.

THE BREAST IMPLANT CONTROVERSY well illustrates many of the points I have been discussing. Although there was almost no reliable scientific information at the time of the ban, several research studies on the subject have been published since then. What sorts of studies were these and what has been learned from them? Before answering these questions, it may be useful to review what was understood even before the research was undertaken, because this influenced the kinds of studies that were done. From the start it was clear that implants could not be the sole cause of connective tissue disease, even if they played some role, since women without breast implants also develop these diseases. And it was also known that breast implants do not invariably cause connective tissue disease, since most women with implants remain healthy. Thus, the most that could have been true is that breast implants *contribute* to connective tissue disease—that is, they might have been a "risk factor" (something that increases the chances of developing a disease). Whether a risk factor is one of several possible causes of a disease or whether it is merely correlated with a real cause may not be known. For this reason, scientists often say that a risk factor is "associated" with a disease, not that it "causes" it.

Risk factors can be strong or weak. For example, cigarette smoking is a strong risk factor for lung cancer. This means that smokers have a very much higher chance of getting lung cancer than nonsmokers. The more they smoke, the greater the risk. In fact, people are extremely unlikely to get lung cancer unless they do smoke. Cigarette smoking is so strong a risk factor for lung cancer that we are justified in saying it "causes" cancer, even though we do not yet know exactly how it does so. In contrast, alcohol may be a weak risk factor for breast cancer. The chances of a drinker getting breast cancer, according to some studies, are slightly higher than the chances of a nondrinker, but abstaining from alcohol is unlikely to confer much protection. It is difficult to prove that something is a risk factor, unless it is a very strong one. The ideal way, scientifically, to prove that something is a risk factor for a particular disease would be to get a large group of very similar people and assign half of them (by random draw) to be exposed to the risk factor and the other half not to be exposed. We would then compare what happens to the two groups. Obviously, we can't do this with breast implants. Women are not likely to volunteer to get breast implants by random draw. Even if such women could be found, it would be unethical to exploit them in this way. So we're left with attempts to get at the same information in less than scientifically ideal ways.

This is where observational epidemiologic studies come in. In this type of study—an increasingly important way of studying connections between disease and potential risk factors—we do not assign people to be exposed to a potential risk. Instead, we observe what happens in those who choose to be exposed for their own reasons or who happen to be exposed inadvertently. Then we compare the incidence of the disease in these people with the incidence in those who are not exposed. There are several forms of observational epidemiologic studies, but only two are of much value in demonstrating risk factors—cohort studies ("cohort" simply means group) and case-control studies. A cohort study of the possible link between breast implants and connective tissue disease would start with a group of women who have implants and a group who do not, none of whom has connective tissue disease. Researchers would then keep track of the two groups over time to see how many in each group develop connective tissue disease. If more in the implant group get a connective tissue disease, it would support (but not prove) the hypothesis that breast implants are a risk factor. In contrast, a case-control study would start with a group of women who already had connective tissue disease (cases) and a group who did not (controls). After the groups were assembled, the researchers would find out how many women in each group had implants. If more cases than controls had breast implants, it would support (but not prove) the hypothesis that breast implants are a risk factor. In either type of study, the bigger the difference between the two groups, the more likely it is that implants are a risk factor. The trickiest part of epidemiologic studies is making sure that the groups are similar to each other in all ways except the possible risk factor (in cohort studies) or the disease (in case-control studies). If they aren't, differences may show up because of other factors (termed "confounding variables").[5]

Cohort and case-control studies each have advantages and disadvantages, but one or the other is necessary to come close to answering the question of whether breast implants are a risk factor for disease. Just finding instances of women with implants who develop connective tissue disease is not enough to prove a connection, because we have to know whether such instances are more common than in women who do not have implants. After all, connective tissue disease might well occur in some people with implants simply by coincidence. Nor can we rely on animal studies, since animals may differ in relevant ways from people. Other laboratory studies are also unable to answer the question of whether breast implants cause connective tissue disease. However, these studies can provide ancillary evidence that an association seen in epidemiologic studies really represents cause and effect. In addition, once a link between a risk factor and a disease is established, laboratory studies or studies of individual patients may be necessary to tell us how the connection works. But they cannot establish the link in the first place. The only way to get at the answer in the implant case is by comparison of women with and without implants (in a cohort study) or by comparion of women with and without connective tissue disease (in a case-control study).

Even though the only way to find out whether breast implants are associated with connective tissue disease is through observational epidemiologic studies, the first reliable one was not published until June 16, 1994.[6] As noted before, this was over two years after breast implants were taken off the market and two months after a class-action settlement was negotiated.

The study, done at the Mayo Clinic and published in the *New England Journal of Medicine,* was a retrospective cohort study, which means that it compared women who had received implants years ago with similar women who had not. The group with implants consisted of all 749 women living in Olmsted County, Minnesota (the location of the Mayo Clinic), who had received breast implants between 1964 and 1991. The group without implants consisted of 1,498 of their neighbors, matched for age. (This control group was selected to minimize confounding variables, such as geographic location or type of medical care. The two groups were similar to each other, except for implants.) The researchers found that the implant group was no more likely to develop connective tissue disease (or related symptoms and abnormal blood tests) than the group without implants. This was not the final word, of course. It was only one study, and it was not large enough to rule out some increase in risk. But it was highly important, because it cast doubt on the whole theory of a link between breast implants and connective tissue disease at a time when many people assumed the theory had been proven. Plaintiffs' attorneys did not like this message, and immediately began a campaign to discredit the messengers. More about that later.

At the time the Mayo Clinic study was published, several other epidemiologic studies were under way. Two were huge, and targeted all connective tissue diseases and a variety of other complaints. The largest was a retrospective cohort study of roughly 400,000 American women in the health professions, about 11,000 of whom had breast implants. This study, called the Women's Health Cohort Study, was published in early 1996 in the *Journal of the American Medical Association.*[7] It found a slight increase in reports of connective tissue disease among women with breast implants. Unfortunately, the authors did not attempt to verify the diagnoses by examining medical records. Since the survey was done after the 1992 FDA ban and the resultant publicity and legal activity, it is difficult to know how much to rely on these self-reports. The authors intend to try to validate the diagnoses in the next phase of the study. Another large retrospective cohort study, published in the *New England Journal of Medicine* in June 1995, could find no association between implants and connective tissue disease in nearly 90,000 nurses, of whom 1,183 had breast implants.[8] An advantage of the Mayo Clinic study and the Nurses' Health Study is that they validated the diagnoses by reviewing medical records. They also investigated a whole range of abnormalities, in addition to well-defined connective tissue diseases. This was to deal with the contention of many people that disease caused by breast implants may not fulfill all the usual criteria of a "classic" connective tissue disease.

Two epidemiologic studies dealt just with scleroderma. Scleroderma, a disease characterized by extensive hardening and scarring of the skin and sometimes of internal organs (in which case it is called systemic sclerosis), is the connective tissue disease most closely linked by anecdotes to silicone breast implants. Neither of the studies[9] could find an association between breast implants and scleroderma. Studies of only rheumatoid arthritis and lupus also did not show an association with implants. Since 1994, then, several epidemiologic studies have failed to find a clear link between breast implants and connective tissue disease.[10]

Does this mean that breast implants do not contribute to connective tissue disease? Not exactly. As explained above, no study can absolutely prove that. All it can do is tell us how likely or unlikely it is. Each study that fails to find a link adds to the evidence that there is none. But since each of them is based on only a sample of women, it is possible to miss a connection. Only if we studied all women with and without implants—an impossible job—could we know for certain whether implants are a risk factor for connective tissue disease. The study of a representative sample simply yields an approximation. There are, fortunately, statistical means for calculating the margin of error, which depends on the size of the sample as well as on the size of any real risk. In the Mayo Clinic study, for example, although no connection was found between implants and connective tissue disease, the study sample was not large enough to rule out with reasonable certainty as much as a threefold increased risk. As other studies are added to the evidence, however, the conclusion that there is no connection grows stronger. The only study that found a connection is difficult to interpret because of the likely bias in self-reports after the FDA ban. Considering all the research together, any risk would have to be very small. Nevertheless, it is still possible that breast implants may cause connective tissue disease in a few women or contribute to it slightly in others. Without an impossibly large study, we may never know.

GIVEN THE FACT that well-designed epidemiologic studies have failed to detect an increased risk of connective tissue disease in women with breast implants, where did the notion come from in the first place? Probably from a combination of anecdotes and speculation that tended to amplify one another. First, there were the poorly documented Japanese reports about direct injections, beginning with a 1964 paper reporting two cases of connective-tissue-like disorders in women who had undergone direct injections of paraffin many years before.[11] (Ironically, this was published at about the time that implants were beginning to replace direct injections in this country.) The disorders did not fall into the usual categories of connective tissue disease, and so the authors of this paper termed them "human adjuvant disease," because they thought the symptoms resembled a disorder of rats injected with a foreign protein combined with an adjuvant (an adjuvant is a substance that enhances an immune response to something else). Later, similar cases were reported in American scientific journals, but these, too, involved direct injections of paraffin or silicone, not the new gel-filled prostheses.[12] It was not until the 1982 Australian publication, mentioned in Chapter 3, that connective tissue disease was reported in women who had silicone-gel-filled breast implants.[13]

Although some still use the term "human adjuvant disease," it has fallen into disrepute, in large part because of the vagueness and variability of the reported signs and symptoms. The problem of vague or shifting definitions of disease continues to plague the study of breast implants. When a study fails to find an increased risk of certain diseases or symptoms in women with implants, adherents of the theory that implants cause disease are quick to suggest that the diseases in question are different. It is impossible to study whether something causes illness, however, unless the illness is clearly described. Otherwise, it cannot be consistently diagnosed and its relation to breast implants cannot be examined. This sort of situation is what Karl Popper, the philosopher of science, had in mind when he said that a scientific hypothesis had to be "falsifiable" to be meaningful. The hypothesis that breast implants cause an undefined set of symptoms is neither provable nor falsifiable—it is simply an assertion.

The idea that breast augmentation caused connective tissue disease had a superficial plausibility. Since local scarring is inevitable in women with breast augmentation, particularly in those who had direct injections, and scarring is also a fea-

ture of certain connective tissue diseases, particularly scleroderma, many people were drawn to the theory that they were
connected. As the isolated reports became the basis of lawsuits
and the publicity grew, more women came forward with similar complaints. Altogether, there are now a few hundred published reports of connective-tissue-like diseases (most without
a clear-cut diagnosis) following breast implants, including the
initial Japanese cases. But there is no way of saying how many
more such cases there are or whether the concurrence in
these women was due to chance alone. Since the ban, women
with implants who are ill are likely to come to attention because of the increased awareness of the problem. This extra
attention may add to the impression that there is a link even
if there isn't. In addition, certain doctors develop a reputation
for believing in a connection, and they may be magnets for patients with breast implants and connective tissue disease or a
variety of symptoms. Studying such women, however, does not
speak to the question of whether implants increase the risk of
disease. The tendency of women with implants and disease to
come forward and the tendency of doctors to study these
women without comparing them with other women can
greatly bias the picture. The possibility of bias underscores why
cohort or case-control studies are so important. Anecdotes
and clinical experience simply can't tell us very much about
the relation between implants and disease. But it is very easy
to believe that they do. A frequent consultant to plaintiffs' attorneys, Frank Vasey, M.D., illustrates the problems with relying on uncontrolled observations. Vasey, the chief of the Division of Rheumatology at the University of South Florida
College of Medicine, became convinced, apparently largely on
the basis of his and others' clinical experience, that breast implants cause disease. In a 1993 book he asserted, "The most
serious conditions that result from the diffusion of silicone

into the body are autoimmune disorders, whereby the body's immune system mistakenly and unceasingly attacks healthy cells, tissues, and musculoskeletal structures."[14] In his view it was confirmatory that 23 of 33 of his patients whose breast implants were removed felt better. But this is precisely the sort of situation in which a powerful placebo effect could operate on both doctor and patient.

A completely different type of research is directed at the question of whether silicone can cause an immune reaction, just as viruses or injected serum can. This line of inquiry assumes that breast implants are risky and seeks to determine the mechanism by which they cause harm. Substances that elicit an immune reaction are called "antigens," which the body combats by forming "antibodies" and special white cells. If silicone elicits an immune reaction, that would lend credence to the theory that silicone causes autoimmune disease, although it would by no means prove it. Many believers in the autoimmune theory are influenced by the presence of inflammation around implants. Some of them mistakenly assume that this is evidence of an immune reaction. In fact, any foreign object embedded in the body elicits inflammation, as explained in Chapter 2. Inflammation does not mean that there is an immune reaction against the object, much less an autoimmune reaction against one's own body. Nevertheless, a similar process in four dogs that Dow Corning used for its experiments elicited a great deal of concern when the company's records were made public, because many people assumed that the inflammation reflected an immune reaction.[15] Believers in the autoimmune theory may also be influenced by the fact that silica (a dust that is the cause of silicosis in miners) is associated in epidemiologic studies with a high incidence of autoimmune disease. But silica dust is different from silicone (although a different type of silica is a constituent of the silicone envelope). The weight of evidence indicates that silicone probably is not capable of acting as an antigen and causing an immune reaction. Nor is there evidence that women with breast implants are more likely to have antibodies against their own tissues (autoantibodies).

One of the adherents of the view that silicone can produce autoimmune disease is Nir Kossovsky, M.D., an assistant professor of pathology at the UCLA Medical Center. He postulates that leaking silicone alters native molecules with which it comes in contact, and forms a complex with them. The body no longer recognizes the altered molecules as native, and mounts an immune reaction against the complex (which serves as the antigen). The reaction then spreads to other parts of the body, where molecules were not altered by contact with silicone. According to Kossovsky, this leads to autoimmune disease. (Autoimmunity refers to a mechanism; connective tissue disease refers to a clinical effect, such as arthritis. Not all connective tissue diseases are known to have an autoimmune basis, but some do and it is strongly suspected in others.) To buttress the theory, Kossovsky has shown that guinea pigs will develop antibodies against silicone-serum complexes, although not to silicone itself. It is quite a leap from these observations to proof of the whole theory that silicone causes autoimmune disease in women with implants. Kossovsky also measured antibodies to fibrinogen (a protein in the blood) and collagen in women with and without implants, some of whom were sick and others of whom were not. He claimed to find higher levels in the sick women with implants, but his methods of analysis have been sharply criticized. In any case, the significance of such a finding is unclear.[16]

Another person who is convinced that silicone causes autoimmune disease is Marc Lappé, formerly a professor of health policy and ethics at the University of Illinois School of Pharmacy. Lappé has a Ph.D. in experimental pathology. He believes that silicone triggers an intense overstimulation of the immune system, perhaps in response to the silica component of the silicone envelope. Lappé published his theory in a journal called *Medical Hypotheses*. It is an interesting theory, but he has produced no persuasive evidence to support it.[17] Like Kossovsky, Lappé is a frequent expert witness or consultant for plaintiffs' attorneys.

It is a long way from such theories to showing that implants cause connective tissue disease. Kossovsky's observations, for example, focus on one link in a long chain of postulated events. But before focusing on one link in a chain of possible causation, scientists usually first try to establish a connection between one end of the chain and the other—that is, between the suspected cause and the disease. For example, first we found out that cigarette smoking is associated with lung cancer. Only then did scientists turn their attention to how cigarettes might cause the disease. (Is it the nicotine or the tars? How does it work? What can we learn from experiments in animals?) In the breast implant controversy, there has been a tendency to do it backwards. Assuming there is a connection, some people have sought to explain how it works. This backwards approach does not invalidate the observations, of course. But it is an inefficient way to address a problem, and it raises the question of bias. The British Department of Health in 1994 issued a thorough review of all the published studies of the immunologic effects of breast implants, and pronounced most of the work "disappointingly poor."[18]

BEFORE LEAVING the subject of scientific research, let me give a brief summary of the salient points I have tried to make. First, a scientific theory must be tested before it can be accepted. Some theories cannot be tested and therefore belong to the realm of assertion, not science. In the breast implant case, the theory that implants cause undefined diseases cannot be tested. It will remain simply a matter of speculation until those attached to the theory describe the symptoms in a way that permits the condition to be consistently diagnosed. No one can study a disease that is not defined or whose definition shifts.

Once a testable hypothesis is proposed, research studies must be designed that speak directly to the hypothesis. In the breast implant case, the hypothesis that implants increase the risk of connective tissue disease requires certain types of epidemiologic studies. The conclusions of a study must be supported by the data and not go beyond the data. For example, in the Mayo Clinic study, the researchers concluded that they could not find an association between implants and the diseases and symptoms they studied. If they had said that implants do not cause connective tissue disease, they would have gone beyond what their data could support. The study did not rule out a connection.

Even well-done scientific studies, appropriately interpreted, produce only probabilistic and tentative answers. There are too many pitfalls in science to embrace any one study uncritically. Researchers make mistakes, some of which are not discovered even with rigorous peer review. Misleading results can also occur just by chance. Each study should therefore be considered a part of a mosaic of information that taken together yields the answer to a scientific question. Of all the properties of scientific research that I have discussed, the most important is the dependence on evidence. No scientific conclusion can be accepted without evidence. This is perhaps the only feature of science that is absolute.

At the time of the ban on breast implants, David Kessler acknowledged that there was no evidence that breast implants cause connective tissue disease. He simply felt he could not wait for the evidence to be assembled before banning them. For their part, the courts had long since decided that implants cause connective tissue disease. Now, years later, the evidence is beginning to emerge. We are beginning to see that any connection between implants and connective tissue disease is likely to be very weak, at most, since several good studies have failed to detect it. Given the absence of scientific evidence at the time, why were the courts so sure of their conclusions?

6

SCIENCE IN THE COURTROOM: OPINIONS WITHOUT EVIDENCE

Dow's conduct in exposing thousands of women to a painful and debilitating disease, and the evidence that Dow gained financially from its conduct, may properly be considered in imposing an award of punitive damages.

—Judge Procter Hug,
August 26, 1994

As we have seen, Maria Stern and her lawyer, Nancy Hersh (with Dan Bolton's help), were the first to go for the legal brass ring by alleging that implants cause connective tissue disease. Stern's disease was never clearly defined in the media, although some press reports referred to it as "arthritis." Until this case, product liability suits against breast implant manufacturers, of which there was a small trickle, had been limited to settlements of no more than $15,000 to $20,000 for local complications.[1] With the 1984 Stern case, all that changed. It was inevitable that after Stern there would be more such cases. After all, many women had connective tissue disease (about 1 in 100) and many had breast implants (also about 1 in 100). Thus, one could expect—on the basis of chance alone—that about 10,000 of the roughly 100 million adult women in the United States would have both.

Once it got out that a link between the two conditions had been accepted in court, women who had both implants and connective tissue disease would be bound to consider whether they, too, should sue. Even those who only thought they might have connective-tissue-like disease also began to take notice. For any who lagged behind, there was plenty of encouragement from many plaintiffs' attorneys.

The issue in the Stern case, as would be true of any product liability suit, was whether the manufacturer of the implants (Dow Corning, in this case) had sold her a defective product that caused her harm. To make the case required that Stern demonstrate two conditions: first, that she was harmed, and second, that the harm was most likely caused by the implants. In addition to demonstrating these conditions, which would satisfy the standard known as "strict liability," there was the question of negligence. Was the manufacturer guilty of knowingly or heedlessly selling a dangerous product? To show negligence required that a third condition be demonstrated—that the manufacturer knew or should have known that the implants were harmful. Theoretically, the first two of these conditions must be met for any product liability suit to be successful. That is theory. In practice, as we shall see, a product liability suit can be spectacularly successful without any of the conditions being fulfilled.

Conditions two and three depend on the satisfaction of the one before it. The manufacturer cannot be held negligent if the implants didn't cause the harm, and the implants cannot be blamed if there is no harm. In most of the breast implant cases that have been brought to trial (but not necessarily in the far more numerous cases settled out of court), the plaintiff has been clearly ill. (In the Stern case, because the records were sealed as a part of an out-of-court settlement after the verdict, it is difficult to be certain about the nature of her medical problems.) The major job of the plaintiff's attorney, therefore, has not been to show that the plaintiff is ill, but to show that the illness was caused by the implants. To do so requires convincing the jury by a "preponderance of the evidence." This is a more relaxed standard than the requirement in a criminal case that the verdict be "beyond a reasonable doubt." But aside from its relative liberality, the phrase "preponderance of the evidence" tells us less than it might seem. It suggests confusingly that there are two kinds of medical evidence—evidence for and evidence against a causal relationship. In practice, this is highly unlikely: either there is evidence for a relationship or there isn't. In the absence of such evidence, the default position must be that there is no link. The burden of proof is on those who assert the relationship.

Sometimes the phrase "preponderance of the evidence" is translated to mean that the jury finds the disease more likely than not to be caused by the breast implants. Or sometimes the same concept is expressed by saying that the breast implants contributed more than 50 percent to the causation of the disease—that is, but for the implants, the disease would not have developed.[2] While neither of these alternative formulations is entirely satisfying, they are an improvement over the vague term "preponderance of the evidence." Furthermore, they can be translated into epidemiologic terms. If connective tissue disease in a typical woman with implants is more likely than not to be caused by implants, it follows that in a large population of women, the majority of cases of connective tissue disease would be due to breast implants. In other words, this cause would have to outweigh all other contributing causes put together. To outweigh all other causes means that women with implants would have to be at least twice as likely to develop the disease as women without implants. (As we saw in the preceding chapter, there is no evidence that they do.)

Notice that what is at issue here is not how certain we are of the effect of implants, but how big the effect is. The degree of certainty is an entirely different matter. I mention the distinction, because some legal scholars confuse the concepts of the size of the effect (as, for example, when it is said that implants contribute more than 50 percent to the disease) with the degree of confidence we can have that it is true. For a scientific finding to be accepted, it is customary to require a 95 percent probability that it is not due to chance alone (I am here giving a shorthand version of a much more complicated statistical concept). Comparing the size of an effect with the probability that a given finding isn't due to chance is comparing apples and oranges. It would be possible to find a huge effect with a low degree of certainty, or a tiny effect with a high degree of certainty. The distinction between the size of an effect and the probability that a particular finding is not due to chance is important in debates about science in the courtroom. It is sometimes said that the reason plaintiffs in court may be awarded damages without good scientific evidence is that the legal standard is more liberal than the scientific standard. According to this argument, all the plaintiff has to do is show preponderance of the evidence, whereas science requires 95 percent confidence about a finding. Not only does this argument confuse size with certainty, but it also confuses the whole with the part. The degree of certainty scientists require refers to the results of a given study, not to a limitless body of evidence. The fundamental issue in both science and the courtroom should be the same—that is, the quality of the evidence. Can we rely on it?

So far, I have been speaking mainly about populations. But courtroom trials are not about populations, they are about individuals. The question is whether breast implants caused disease in *this* woman. Is there any basis for such a judgment? I do not believe there is. Given the absence of any scientific information on individual differences in women's responses to breast implants, we can only look at the individual as an *average* woman with implants. We have no basis, at least in the current state of knowledge, for making a judgment about a particular woman. We therefore *must* appeal to epidemiologic data—that is, to studies of populations. We have to assume that whatever is true on average is true of the particular woman. As it happens, we think this way intuitively. When we wonder whether someone we know developed lung cancer because he smokes, we automatically consider what we know about the risks of smoking in a population. We can't be sure that cigarette smoking caused disease in this particular man, because there is no test to answer that question in his case, but we think it probably did because we know a lot about the risks of smoking in populations. Without considering what we know about populations, we have no basis for our opinion. Despite our intuitive realization that particular cases must be considered in the light of what we know about the general situation, that is not what juries are instructed to do. They are asked to judge the particular case on the basis of the evidence presented in court, and no matter how unsatisfactory that evidence is, they must reach a verdict. They cannot say, as scientists can, that they will not form an opinion until they get more or better evidence.

Science in the courtroom is paradoxical in that it always yields a firm conclusion, yet never does. Each plaintiff who claims that breast implants caused her connective tissue disease requires a verdict, and a verdict is always reached. But even though the issue is settled for the last plaintiff, it is not settled for the next one. The question must be revisited over and over, for every woman who comes to court claiming a connection. Even so, it is not argued completely from scratch. An earlier verdict for a plaintiff provides a powerful presumption in the next case (for technical reasons, a verdict for a defendant does not). Nevertheless, verdicts can differ, no matter how similar the women's cases. In contrast, scientists almost never claim to have settled a "case." Their findings are conditional. More work is nearly always required. But for any one scientific question, the weight of the accumulated evidence tends to converge toward an answer. Eventually the probability of the answer will be great enough to warrant general acceptance of the conclusion.

In product liability cases, expert testimony by scientists is usually central. The question of causation is, after all, a scientific one. But scientific questions are handled very differently in the courtroom than they are outside the courtroom. The difference turns on the relationship between evidence and opinion. In both science and law, of course, "expert" opinion is important. But what that means in the two professions is as far apart as day and night. As discussed in the preceding chapter, scientists, no matter how expert, must provide the evidence on which their opinions are based. When they complete a research study, it is necessary to present their evidence before their conclusions will be accepted. Even when they are commenting on the general state of their field, it is customary for them to cite explicitly the basis of their opinions. For example, medical researchers sometimes publish summaries of what is already known about a subject. Called "review articles," these summaries are analogous to expert testimony in court, in that they are evaluations of the state of knowledge. But even review articles must refer to the published research being evaluated (unpublished work usually counts for very little in science). In addition, it is expected that authors of review articles will be as even-handed as possible—that is, reasonably comprehensive and unbiased in the selection of the work they discuss. Indeed, an important question for peer reviewers is whether a review article is objective and balanced.

Expert testimony in the courtroom is very different. In contrast to scientific procedures, an expert witness in court is *expected* to give an educated guess, not to produce evidence.[3] Whether expert testimony is admitted in court turns largely on the witness's "credibility"—which means his or her credentials. Does the expert have the appropriate training and experience? Even these rather minimalist standards are often only loosely applied. In the courtroom, one scientist can seem much like another. Some distinctly second-rate scientists testify in trial after trial and consult in case after case, sometimes even earning their living that way. In essence they become well-practiced, professional witnesses, whose major talent is convincing juries, not evaluating evidence. In fact, they may cite no evidence at all, or allude to evidence only vaguely, without giving its source. Sometimes, they refer to their own, unpublished work as evidence, but no one has the opportunity to evaluate its validity or even to know whether it exists. Many reputable scientists refuse to be expert witnesses in court, probably in part because they find the adversarial process an unsatisfactory way to arrive at scientific conclusions and therefore

feel uncomfortable participating in it. Often experts are chosen whose field is not relevant to the scientific question that
needs answering. In many of the breast implant cases, for example, plaintiffs' attorneys have relied on pathologists or tox-
icologists to speculate about how breast implants might cause
connective tissue disease, rather than calling on epidemiologists who would get to the question of whether they actually
do. In the Stern case, for example, her key witnesses consisted
of a pathologist, a toxicologist, and an immunologist.[4] Even
more troubling, expert witnesses are selected by the contest-
ing lawyers, paid by them, and their testimony is rehearsed in
advance—circumstances unlikely to ensure competence, let
alone objectivity. In fact, the whole point is precisely to find a
"qualified" witness who will be scientifically committed to your
side. The irony here is that a lawyer may employ a scientist to
offer eccentric views in a court proceeding that is supposed to
hold manufacturers to generally accepted, mainstream standards.

AFTER CONTRIBUTING so decisively to the handsome verdict in
the Stern case, Dan Bolton was on a roll. He left Hersh and
Hersh and went on to become a partner in another firm and
a magnet for breast implant suits. The decision in Bolton's
next big case—the case of Mariann Hopkins—was appealed
all the way to the Supreme Court, which refused to review it.
In its own way, this case was even more influential than the
Stern case, because it was instrumental in the FDA ban.

Mariann Hopkins, of Sebastopol, California, a secretary
at Sonoma State University in nearby Rehnert Park and the
wife of a San Francisco firefighter, was in her early thirties
when she underwent a double mastectomy in 1976 because of
fibrocystic disease of the breast.[5] This is a very common con-

dition that produces tender nodules in the breasts, particularly just before menstrual periods. Whether it is a precursor of breast cancer or not has been debated for decades. The consensus is that it usually isn't, although some forms of it may increase the risk. In any case, Hopkins evidently did not want to take the chance. After her mastectomy she had her breasts reconstructed with silicone-gel-filled implants, manufactured by Dow Corning. Within a few months, one of them ruptured, and to maintain symmetry she had them both replaced.

Three years later, in 1979, she was told she had an autoimmune disorder called mixed connective tissue disease. This is a devastating disease, with clinical features of systemic lupus, rheumatoid arthritis, polymyositis, and scleroderma, all rolled into one. Typically, the disease produces very high levels of antibodies against constituents of the patient's own cells. Mixed connective tissue disease is incurable, and Hopkins had to be treated indefinitely with corticosteroids, which can produce a variety of serious side effects. In 1986, seven years after the diagnosis, Hopkins gave up her job because of her disabling disease. The same year she again had her breast implants replaced because one had ruptured.

In 1987, Hopkins's mother told her that she had heard there was a link between ruptured breast implants and autoimmune disorders. Hopkins queried her doctors, who told her they knew of no such connection. She later said the rheumatologist who was treating her mixed connective tissue disease, Dr. Stephen Gospe, was "very patronizing. He said people always need something to blame and I might as well accept my illness." The next year, however, Hopkins happened to turn on the evening news as she came into her house from the grocery store and saw a clip of Bolton, along with Sybil Goldrich, talking about the effects of silicone leakage on the immune system. (Goldrich, you will remember, is co-founder of the advocacy group Command Trust Network; Bolton was at the time testifying before the November 1988 FDA advisory panel.) To Hopkins, seeing Bolton on television was little short of a miracle. As she said later, "If I'd turned it on one minute later, I would have missed it." But she didn't miss it, and she straightaway phoned Bolton in San Francisco. Hopkins said of that conversation, "I learned there were other women besides myself who'd had problems with implants. I said 'Why haven't I heard of this?' He said, 'Because there have been suits filed against Dow Corning and they have settled out of court, and then all the documents are kept under lock and key.' " The next month, she and Bolton filed suit against Dow Corning in federal court in San Francisco.[6]

At the trial three years later, in 1991, Bolton called three expert witnesses to testify as to the cause of Hopkins's disease—Marc Lappé, Nir Kossovsky, and Frank Vasey. Because these three, whom I introduced in the preceding chapter, have been so important in breast implant litigation, it is worth examining their credentials in some detail. Lappé, who you may recall from Chapter 5 has a Ph.D. in experimental pathology, testified in the Stern case, as well as the Hopkins case, according to an article in *American Lawyer*.[7] In both cases, his testimony primarily concerned his interpretation of the Dow Corning laboratory studies. In his view Dow Corning's animal studies indicated that breast implants may have contributed to Stern's and Hopkins's illnesses. A 1995 computer search of Lappé's own publications, as compiled by the National Library of Medicine, is revealing. As mentioned earlier, he published his theory about the way in which implants might cause autoimmune disease in an article in the journal *Medical Hypotheses*, confidently titled, "Silicone-Reactive Disorder: A New

Autoimmune Disease Caused by Immunostimulation and Superantigens." As a hypothesis, it contributed no new evidence. In its 1994 review of the scientific evidence in the breast implant controversy, the British Department of Health said Lappé's paper "has nothing to add to the issue of a causal relationship between silicones, immunological responsiveness and disease."[8] Of Lappé's 50-some scientific papers in the National Library of Medicine's database, only one other dealt with the subject of breast implants. (His other papers have dealt mainly with the ethics of genetic screening.) He also published a 1991 book, *Chemical Deception: The Toxic Threat to Health and the Environment.*[9]

Kossovsky is an M.D. certified in anatomic pathology, the study of diseased tissues.[10] An assistant professor at the UCLA Medical Center, he has been a very popular and effective plaintiffs' witness in breast implant cases. At the time of the Hopkins trial, Kossovsky was in his early thirties and looked younger. Pleasantly voluble, with an engaging, eager manner, Kossovsky gives the impression of wanting nothing more than to explain the immune system to the jury. He believes that silicone changes body tissues in such a way that the body no longer recognizes them as native. In its effort to reject what it interprets as "foreign" invaders, the body mounts an autoimmune reaction that leads to connective tissue disease. Despite Kossovsky's long-standing attachment to this theory, there is still no good evidence for it.

Bolton's third witness on causation was Frank Vasey, the chief of the Division of Rheumatology at the University of South Florida College of Medicine.[11] Rheumatology is the medical specialty concerned with connective tissue disease. Vasey, a physician, has reported a group of patients with breast implants who had connective tissue disease or symptoms suggestive of it, most of whom felt better after the implants were removed.[12] In medical practice, it is not unusual for a specialist who attracts patients with a certain type of problem to gain erroneous impressions about its frequency or its association with other conditions. Without controls and appropriate population sampling techniques, it is easy to draw conclusions that will not stand up to later, more careful epidemiologic analysis. Even a large clinical experience, while possibly suggestive, cannot substitute for a cohort or case-control study in getting at whether implants cause disease. The history of medicine is replete with examples of mistaken "clinical impressions" based on uncontrolled and often undocumented personal experience. One of the major advances in modern medicine is the realization that to be reliable, personal experience must be supported by rigorous research.

None of Bolton's witnesses was an epidemiologist. Yet this is the only kind of specialist who could authoritatively speak to the issue of a possible link between breast implants and connective tissue disease.

Perhaps the most startling testimony on the other side was that of Hopkins's own rheumatologist, Stephen Gospe. Gospe had definitively diagnosed Hopkins's mixed connective tissue disease in 1979, but he believed her symptoms began even before she received her first set of implants in 1976. Indeed, because of suggestive symptoms, her internist, Dr. Louis Pelfini, had in 1975 ordered a test for autoimmune disease, which at the time was inconclusive. Because her symptoms persisted, Pelfini sent her to Gospe in 1979. Gospe's testimony that her symptoms had begun before her first implants were placed in 1976 might have been expected to undermine the plaintiff's case. But evidently it didn't trouble the jurors. On December 13, 1991, the jury awarded Hopkins $7.34 million. Dow Corning was found guilty of fraud and malice in marketing the implants.[13] The evidence included the Dow Corning memo instructing salespeople to wash off demonstration implants so that plastic surgeons would not notice the oiliness of the envelope. The Hopkins case reached its climax just as David Kessler was deciding whether to permit implants to stay on the market. This timing, nearly everyone agrees, greatly influenced the FDA's ultimate decision.

Dow Corning (which went out of the implant business a few months after the Hopkins decision)[14] appealed to the U.S. Court of Appeals for the Ninth Circuit. Signaling the significance of the case, two renowned lawyers joined the fray in the appeal. Harvard Law School professor Laurence Tribe headed the Hopkins-Bolton team. Shirley Hufstedler, Jimmy Carter's former secretary of education and a former judge of the Ninth Circuit, joined Frank Woodside III for Dow Corning's defense. The defense's appeal was based on two arguments. The first concerned the statute of limitations, a technical argument of interest to lawyers but probably no one else. The second argument was whether the testimony had established that it was more probable than not that there was a causal connection between Hopkins's breast implants and her mixed connective tissue disease—the second necessary condition for a product liability judgment. The first condition had clearly been met: no one doubted that Hopkins was sick. But the other two conditions were in contention, and the satisfaction of the third (that Dow Corning had been negligent or wanton) was contingent on proving the second (that the implants most likely caused the mixed connective tissue disease). The appellate court was asked to consider whether the lower court had adequate evidence for this finding. And in particular, was it correct in relying on the expert testimony Bolton had assembled?

Dow's Woodside (a physician as well as a lawyer) had argued in lower court that Lappé, Kossovsky, and Vasey were not qualified to testify as experts on causation, but the trial judge had disagreed. The appeal was largely based on the same argument, and again it was dismissed. Although the appeals court noted that scientific testimony must be "not only relevant, but reliable," it ruled that the testimony of Kossovsky, Lappé, and Vasey had met this standard. Kossovsky and Vasey, according to the court, had based their opinions in part on "preliminary results" of epidemiological studies they were conducting. Four years later, in a search of the medical literature, I was unable to find that either of them has published a rigorous epidemiologic study that could shed light on the question of causation. Lappé was said to be "a recognized expert on the immunological effects of silicone in the human body," although a search of the National Library of Medicine's comprehensive database shows that he has published very little on the subject.

Judge Procter Hug, writing for the Court of Appeals, not only accepted the testimony of the three witnesses, but his opinion indicated that he was utterly convinced about the substance of the matter—not just about the procedural questions.[15] He was certain, even if most scientists were not, that breast implants cause mixed connective tissue disease. Referring to the many thousands of women who have Dow Corning implants, the judge said, "Each of these women was at risk of encountering the same fate from which Hopkins suffered." As for Dow Corning, he said, "Dow's conduct in exposing thousands of women to a painful and debilitating disease, and the evidence that Dow gained financially from its conduct, may properly be considered in imposing an award of punitive damages." The harshness of Judge Hug's conclusion reflected the emphasis in the case on the Dow Corning documents. Dow Corning petitioned the U.S. Supreme Court for review. The petition was refused, thus letting stand the appellate court's decision.[16] Bolton's experts had done their job well.

WITH THE ASTONISHING EXPLOSION of scientific knowledge over the last century, and particularly in the last 50 years, expert testimony has become increasingly important in the courts. In particular, there are few product liability suits in which expert testimony is not central. In the *Hopkins* case, for example, the testimony of Lappé, Kossovsky, and Vasey was pivotal. But even as expert testimony became commonplace in the courtroom, legal scholars and judges began to fret about its role. Who was an expert? How should expert testimony be received and what weight should it have? As far back as 1858, the U.S. Supreme Court foresaw the problems in store. It observed then that "experience has shown that opposite opinions of persons professing to be experts may be obtained to any amount," and it went on to complain that cross-examination of all these experts was virtually useless, "wasting the time and wearying the patience of both court and jury, and perplexing, instead of elucidating, the questions involved."[17]

In 1897, possibly because it had heard enough, the Supreme Court decided to cut things short by limiting cross-examination of experts. In considering an insanity defense for a man accused of murder, an expert witness had been asked in lower court, "What does medical science teach as to that?" Incredibly, the witness was told by the trial judge that he didn't have to answer that question. On appeal, the Supreme Court agreed, saying that once an expert gives his opinion, the court should take it or leave it. It would be "opening the door to too wide an inquiry to interrogate him as to what other scientific men [*sic*] have said upon such matters, or in respect to the general teachings of science thereon, or to permit books of science to be offered in evidence." The message, then, was not to delve into something as arcane as scientific evidence. Whatever a qualified witness said was okay.

This decision pretty much settled the issue until a federal trials court in 1923 reached the polar opposite conclusion in *Frye v. United States*. In *Frye*, the issue in contention was whether a "lie detector test" (which in those days was simply a blood pressure reading) would be admitted as evidence. The court refused to admit it, on the grounds that there was not yet a scientific consensus about the validity of this new method. Far from agreeing with the Supreme Court that experts needn't take into account the work of other scientists, the *Frye* court said that testimony *must* speak to the work of others—that is, it was admissible only if it incorporated principles and methods generally accepted by the relevant scientific community. The Court of Appeals agreed. Thus was born the "general acceptance" standard for expert testimony, a subject of intense legal debate for the next 70 years. This standard had the effect of excluding a good deal of what has become known as "junk science"—patently absurd testimony by zealots, incompetents, or opportunists. But the *Frye* standard was by no means accepted in all courts. Its opponents claimed, somewhat improbably, that it would tend to exclude novel, farsighted testimony by modern-day Galileos.[18] There is no record of this happening once, let alone often. Furthermore, even if a modern-day Galileo did not make it into court at first, that fact would not stop him from prevailing in the scientific community. Courts do not determine scientific acceptance, as implied by the argument that we need to keep our courts open to the hidden Galileos in our midst.

What the don't-ask-don't-tell approach of the 1897 Supreme Court had in common with the *Frye* decision was that both avoided coming to grips with the substantive issue of how to define good scientific evidence that would qualify for admissibility in court. *Frye* evaded the issue by setting up a proxy, and a very good proxy it was: Good science was determined by other scientists through their usual methods—peer review and publication, criticism, replication—and, most important, by its reliability in predicting future results. (These were not the words of *Frye*, but they are its effect.) In 1975 new Federal Rules of Evidence were signed into law by President Ford. These detailed rules for admitting evidence into federal courts contain criteria for scientific testimony that include validity but omit the requirement for general acceptance in the scientific community. Whether the new, more liberal Rules superseded *Frye* or not was not clear. Some courts went with *Frye*, others with the Rules, and others simply followed their own instincts. The courts thus continued their chaotic approach to the problem, even while product liability suits were burgeoning and scientists themselves were having a difficult time keeping up with the rapid advances in their own fields.

In 1993 the U.S. Supreme Court finally grasped the nettle and attempted to deal substantively with the problem of expert testimony in the courts. The case that occasioned the Supreme Court's attention, *Daubert v. Merrell Dow Pharmaceuticals*, was in many respects similar to the breast implant cases.[19] The case was brought against Merrell Dow Pharmaceuticals in 1984 by the parents of two boys who had been born with only rudimentary arms, a well-known congenital mishap (these sorts of defects occur in about 1 in 1,000 births). The parents alleged that the defect had been caused by Merrell Dow's Bendectin, an antihistamine-like drug that the two mothers had taken during pregnancy to combat morning sickness. Bendectin was an extraordinarily popular drug, prescribed for pregnant women almost as routinely as vitamins. Some 17 million women took it (as did I) between 1958 and 1983. It is not surprising, then, that even if there were no connection, babies with upper-limb defects would sometimes be born to mothers who had taken Bendectin, just as connective tissue disease would sometimes develop in women who had breast implants even if there were no causal connection between the implants and the disease.

Merrell Dow's Frank Woodside (who would later be Dow Corning's attorney in the Hopkins case) had argued at first that the case should not be tried at all. He pointed out that there had been many epidemiologic studies published in the scientific literature, involving some 130,000 women, none of which had been able to show a connection between Bendectin and birth defects. The plaintiffs, however, produced eight expert witnesses who testified to Bendectin's ability to cause birth defects, although they could point to no epidemiologic evidence. One witness testified that she had reanalyzed the published studies that Woodside cited and had come to the opposite conclusion, although she had not published her work. The trial court, citing *Frye,* agreed that the plaintiffs had produced no admissible evidence. The appeals court agreed. The Supreme Court was then asked to speak to the narrow issue of whether *Frye* was the approriate standard or whether it had been superseded by the 1975 Rules of Evidence. Merrell Dow favored *Frye,* since it had worked well for them, but the plaintiffs wanted the less stringent Federal Rules of Evidence to prevail.

The Supreme Court dispensed quickly with the narrow question. Yes, the Federal Rules did supersede *Frye,* and the case was passed back to the appeals court to hear again under those rules. The Supreme Court made no attempt to decide whether Bendectin caused birth defects, only what the standards for the admissibility of expert evidence should be. But the Court also devoted considerable attention to elucidating the meaning of those standards and how they were to be applied, thus finally dealing with the issue of what constitutes good science. A large number of interested individuals and organizations, including the *New England Journal of Medicine*, were aware of the enormous impact the *Daubert* decision might have. The Court was therefore flooded with amici briefs on both sides. These revealed interesting schisms within the scientific community. Many favored the *Frye* standard (as did we), because they felt it would reduce the amount of junk science finding its way to the courts. We argued that testimony should be based on research that had been duly published in peer-reviewed journals. But equally reputable scientists came down on the other side, because they felt the "general acceptance" criterion was too restrictive and elitist. And many lawyers also opposed the *Frye* standard because they believed it would preempt the responsibility of juries to decide the facts.

In the end both sides in the *Daubert* case claimed victory— or defeat, depending on whether one is inclined to see the glass as half full or half empty. The Supreme Court said that while the Federal Rules applied, this did not mean that all expert testimony would be admissible. Far from it. Federal judges are now required to undertake "a preliminary assessment of whether the reasoning or methodology underlying the testimony is scientifically valid and of whether that reasoning or methodology properly can be applied to the fact in issue." Thus, judges are to be the gatekeepers who decide whether to admit expert testimony. This was not what either side thought they wanted. The *Frye* proponents wanted the scientific community to be gatekeepers. The other side didn't want any gatekeepers; let the juries decide on the basis of the cross-examination. But in *Daubert*, the Supreme Court said that judges must decide, and they must do so by learning how to think like scientists. Expert testimony must be both "reliable" and "relevant," and judges should decide in advance whether it was. Writing for the majority, Justice Harry Blackmun emphasized the importance of relevance by pointing out that testimony about the effect of the phases of the moon on irrational behavior might be quite valid as to the astronomical data, but totally irrelevant in drawing any inference about behavior. What is relevant in one context may not be in another. This requirement that expert testimony be apposite to the matter at hand was at issue in the appeal of the *Hopkins* decision.

Many concerned about the increasingly contentious relations between law and science welcomed the *Daubert* decision. Bert Black, a lawyer and then-chair of the American Bar Association's Standing Committee on Scientific Evidence, and Francisco Ayala, a scientist and then-president of the American Association for the Advancement of Science, together with a colleague, Carol Saffran-Brinks, wrote a celebratory analysis in the *Texas Law Review*.[20] Despite the fact that both Black and Ayala had participated in an amicus brief on behalf of Merrell Dow—technically the losing side—they saw the actual written judgment as a cause for hope that the days of junk science in the courtroom were numbered. In particular, they approved of the sophisticated analysis of what good science is. The Supreme Court embraced the notion of Karl Popper, the philosopher of science, that good science requires formulating a question that can be answered. In other words, any hypothesis must be capable of being tested. It is useless to come up with a theory, no matter how plausible, that cannot be proved or disproved. Black and his colleagues, in a section on the "pathological science" that stems from ignoring the necessity for testing and corroboration, describe it as "characterized by a fixation on effects that are difficult to detect, a readiness to disregard prevailing ideas and theories, and an unwillingness to conduct meaningful experimental testing." This description is relevant in the breast implant controversy. The common contention that breast implants cause diseases that cannot be objectively described is a theory that cannot be tested. Doctors who believe in it simply assert that such diseases exist and that they know them when they see them.

For those who might have thought the Supreme Court's *Daubert* decision heralded a new, more rational era in the courts, let alone mere consistency, subsequent events are instructive. The Supreme Court decided the *Daubert* case in 1993, sending it back to the Ninth Circuit Appeals Court for reconsideration. By coincidence, this was the same court that considered the appeal in the Hopkins case in 1994. The *Daubert* decision was handed down after the Hopkins verdict but before the appeal. A major issue in the petition to the U.S. Supreme Court was the failure of the Ninth Circuit Appeals Court to adhere to the *Daubert* criteria. As we have seen, the appellate court found the expert testimony in Hopkins admissible, even though its decision was handed down after the *Daubert* decision. Just a year later, however, the same court found that the testimony that Bendectin caused birth defects was *not* admissible.[21] I believe that in *neither* case had the testimony clearly met the Supreme Court's requirement for reliability and relevance. Even more difficult to comprehend is the fact that the Supreme Court itself, after its insightful analysis of good science in *Daubert* in 1993, let stand the Hopkins decision in 1995. (If you are having trouble following all this, it is not your fault, or even mine.) The inconsistency of the decisions surely underscores the continuing confusion about what kind of scientific evidence should be admitted in court. The *Daubert* decision doesn't seem to have helped much, at least not yet.

As I have noted, scientific testimony in the courtroom is often at most only marginally related to scientific evidence. To be sure, there are superficial matters of form that may suggest a resemblance between science in and out of the courtroom. Expert witnesses may wear white coats, be called "doctor," purport to do research, and talk scientific jargon. But too often they are merely adding a veneer to a foregone, self-interested conclusion. Sometimes they spin theories that they say are supported by their expertise or experience. Or they may refer vaguely to research. Very often, however, the "research" is their own and it is unpublished and unavailable. The point is that they are not required to produce their evidence, and they usually do not. The result is a growing gap between scientific reality and what passes for it in the courtroom. The *Daubert* decision was a brave step toward remedying the situation, but it was not enough. In Chapter 10, I will discuss other solutions.

7

GREED AND CORRUPTION: ALL THAT FREE MONEY

Q: Your family wants you to take the money and run?
A: I think so.

—Healthy woman with implants interviewed on
KHOU-TV, Houston,
October 10, 1994

A ny moralist who wanted to preach about the corrupting effects of money could find no better parable than the story of silicone breast implants. The lure of money permeates all aspects of the saga. It goes without saying that the manufacturers and plastic surgeons had financial interests in maintaining that the implants were safe—even when they didn't know whether that was true. What is far less obvious are the outsized interests of the other players—the plaintiffs' and defense lawyers, the doctors who diagnose and treat women with breast implants, the witnesses and consultants who sell their expertise for around $500 hourly,[1] and the women with breast implants who are most probably not sick but will not pass up the opportunity to gain from the dispute. As billions of dollars change hands, we should remember where the money originates. It comes from consumers who buy any of the goods made by breast implant manufacturers or by other manufacturers who are insured for liability costs by the same insurors. Whenever a consumer purchases a Corning Ware dish, for example, he or she also pays a "tort tax." Case by case, settlement by settlement, the billions of dollars collected in this way are transferred to the plaintiffs, their lawyers, and the doctors and scientists who help them, as well as the inevitable administrative apparatus that oversees the transfer.

Sometimes the transfer of funds from manufacturer to plaintiff and lawyer occurs in large, seemingly arbitrary chunks. The best example is the $25 million verdict awarded in 1992 to Pamela Johnson of Houston.[2] This verdict eclipsed the record $7.34 million awarded to Mariann Hopkins. Paradoxically, despite the size of the verdict, the Johnson case was weak. Pamela Johnson, a forty-six-year-old administrative assistant, claimed that when one of her breast implants ruptured, the silicone gel released into her tissues caused her to become ill. The nature of the illness was not clear. According to her lawyer, she had a silicone-induced "autoimmune disorder, in which she feels like she has a bad case of the flu all the time." But she had apparently not been diagnosed as having any well-recognized immune disorder or connective tissue disease. Instead, she had a variety of vague, nonspecific complaints, such as recurrent sinusitis, sore throats, colds, and bladder infections.[3] Thus, this case did not clearly fulfill even the first of the usual conditions for a product liability suit, since the medical harm suffered by Pamela Johnson was nebulous.

With the Johnson case, the center of breast implant litigation shifted from San Francisco to Houston, where John O'Quinn, of the law firm O'Quinn, Kerensky & McAninch, quickly established himself as the plaintiffs' attorney who could make the most from the least. His tactic was to glide over the issue of whether Johnson was sick, and concentrate instead on her concern that she *might* get sick. He also seized every opportunity to shift the jury's focus from Johnson to all the other women with breast implants. He suggested that Johnson was somehow a proxy for these other women, all of whom shared fears engendered by the implants—certainly a self-fulfilling prophecy, if ever there was one.

Johnson had breast implants for augmentation in 1976, the year implants came under the purview of the FDA. At the time she was twenty-nine years old. The implants were made by Medical Engineering Corporation (MEC), later a subsidiary of Bristol-Myers Squibb. Johnson was apparently fine until 13 years later, when her breasts became hard. She went to see her plastic surgeon, Philip Rothenberg, who performed a closed capsulotomy to break up the scar tissue—despite the fact that the package inserts had for six years (during which Rothenberg performed many implantations) warned that this procedure was known to carry a high risk of rupture. Within a few days, her left breast was swollen and painful. Rothenberg operated, and found, not surprisingly, that her left implant had ruptured. According to the testimony in the trial, Rothenberg found it so difficult to clean out the spilled silicone gel that he had to do a partial mastectomy. He then put in another set of implants, also made by MEC. Unhappy with the appearance of her breasts, Johnson consulted another plastic surgeon, Fabian Worthing, who replaced her implants with a pair made by another manufacturer. Three years later, in 1992 (the year of the FDA ban), she returned to Worthing complaining of fatigue and other vague symptoms that she said doctors had attributed to the implants. Worthing removed them.

O'Quinn had a weak case. Everything depended on creating sympathy for Johnson, on the face of it not an easy prospect. Johnson's implants were cosmetic, which many people frown on. More important, unlike Mariann Hopkins, Johnson did not have a recognized autoimmune or connective tissue disease. Although she spoke tearfully of "sinus infections, sore throat infections, upper respiratory infections, bladder infection . . . one right after the other," this is not usually the stuff of multimillion-dollar suits. The complaints might seem more likely related to her cigarette habit, rather than her breast implants. Furthermore, since Rothenberg may have ruptured her left implant, shouldn't he be the target of the suit? O'Quinn had to convince the jury that the implants had ruptured because they were defective, not because Rothenberg performed a closed capsulotomy. Subtly, O'Quinn shifted the usual burden of proof. Instead of the plaintiff having to show harm, the manufacturers had to show the implants were safe.

There were good, practical reasons for suing the manufacturer rather than the plastic surgeon. First, it is safe to assume that Bristol-Myers Squibb had deeper pockets than Rothenberg. Second, juries are generally less sympathetic to large, impersonal corporations than they are to doctors. Rothenberg had originally been named as a defendant, but Johnson dropped her claim against him before the trial. Rothenberg ultimately testified for Johnson and O'Quinn.

O'Quinn's partner, Richard Laminack, first realized the advantages of suing the manufacturer instead of the plastic surgeon in 1988, when, according to an interview in *Texas Monthly*, a surgeon told him, "I know you're suing me, but I could be your best witness."[4] A case of medical malpractice was thus converted to a product liability case. In Texas, however, it is best to name the surgeon in the suit initially, as well as the manufacturer, then drop the surgeon's name. This maneuver helps to ensure that the case is tried in a state court instead of a federal court. If the surgery was done in the state and the lawsuit includes the surgeon, it is a state case. That is a tremendous advantage in Texas where the courts are notoriously friendly to plaintiffs' attorneys.

The pattern of suing the doctor along with the manufacturer, then dropping the suit against the doctor in return for his or her cooperation, is well recognized in breast implant cases.[5] Helpful doctors can greatly strengthen a plaintiff's case. Implant manufacturers themselves have contributed to the likelihood of the surgeon supporting the plaintiff by refusing to indemnify plastic surgeons when they are sued—in contrast to automobile companies, which routinely indemnify car dealerships for the costs of litigation. This is a very short-sighted economy. The plastic surgeons are then at the mercy of the plaintiffs' attorneys. They can either cooperate with the plaintiff or risk being a target of the suit themselves.

So successful was O'Quinn in the Johnson case that it was the subject of a teaching videotape (Video Trial Report, a joint venture of *American Lawyer* magazine and Courtroom Television Network). Titled "Look Over Here: *Johnson v. Bristol-Myers Squibb Company,*" the tape was subtitled, "How Houston Plaintiff's Lawyer John O'Quinn Won the Largest Breast Implant Verdict to Date by Keeping a Jury on the Strongest Elements of His Case." The narrator makes it clear that O'Quinn had to avoid the issue of whether Johnson was sick and instead concentrate on the possibility that she might in the future become ill because of the silicone in her body. O'Quinn spoke of "all the lymphomas and the cancer and all the real serious diseases of that nature that are found among these hundreds of thousands of women with this condition."

More specifically, he evoked the story of Johnson's mother, who had breast cancer, implying that breast implants might increase Johnson's risk of suffering a similar fate.

O'Quinn's most successful witness was the youthful, ingratiating Nir Kossovsky (whom I introduced in Chapters 5 and 6), by now well experienced in breast implant cases. Using markers and a large pad mounted on a tripod, Kossovsky delivered an eager lesson in immunology, illustrated with drawings of white cells. He showed the white cells taking part in inflammation, which he said could progress to an immune reaction, then an autoimmune reaction—a hypothetical sequence stated as fact. He also said that the sequence could be caused by breast implants, despite the lack of evidence on this point. Quite apart from the unproved assertions in Kossovsky's testimony, it was not at all clear that his theory had anything to do with Johnson. Although the plaintiff's side implied that breast implants had affected Johnson's immune system, it was not claimed that she was suffering from a known autoimmune disease, such as rheumatoid arthritis or systemic lupus erythematosus (diseases Kossovsky himself mentioned when asked for examples of autoimmune disorders). But unless Johnson had an autoimmune disease, it is difficult to understand how Kossovsky's testimony fulfilled the Supreme Court's requirement for relevance.

One of Bristol-Myers Squibb's expert witnesses, Noel Rose, professor of pathology and of molecular microbiology and immunology at Johns Hopkins University and a widely recognized authority on autoimmune diseases, said that on the basis of Johnson's medical records he thought it "highly unlikely" that she had an autoimmune disorder. Yet the narrator of the videotape referred to Rose ironically as "one of the best witnesses for the plaintiff." Perhaps this characterization was partly because of his scholarly mien and cautious answers, which contrasted with Kossovsky's quick certainties. But it was also because when O'Quinn asked Rose whether he could understand the fears of women with silicone in their bodies, Rose answered, "I can imagine how they feel. Of course, I'm not in that position myself." When O'Quinn responded, "You're lucky," Rose answered, "I am indeed." Did Rose mean he was lucky not to be Johnson, or did he mean he was lucky to be Rose? It was impossible to tell. He has since told me he was merely affirming his "sympathy for all of the women who have had breast implants and been told that they have silicone 'time bombs' in their bodies." In any case, this double entendre was apparently all it took to undercut Rose's substantive testimony that Johnson most probably did not have autoimmune disease and that there was no scientific evidence of a connection between breast implants and such diseases, anyway. On such subtle theater turns a $25-million verdict.

The jury in the Johnson case was acting in the generous tradition of juries hearing product liability suits. When a plaintiff seems hurt, vulnerable, and appealing (Johnson was very tearful), and the company is large, anonymous, and impervious, juries are predisposed to even up the score. O'Quinn also was very careful in selecting his jury. He hired consultants from the Wilmington Institute, a jury research organization in Dallas, who studied the attitudes of potential jurors on the breast implant issue and helped to rehearse the testimony. According to the *National Law Journal*, O'Quinn did not accept jurors who were reluctant to award damages for pain and suffering or verdicts larger than $1 million. He was also very watchful for prospective jurors who might be biased against women who had implants for augmentation.[6] O'Quinn is said to be convinced that blue-collar men make ideal jurors in breast implant cases, because they are guilty about pressuring women to acquire large breasts; upper-middle-class white women are the worst, because they are likely to have considered implants, but rejected the idea.[7]

The jury was generous to O'Quinn, as well as to Johnson. His fee was 40 percent of the award (45 percent if there had been an appeal), plus expenses.[8] Although O'Quinn had already established a highly successful career as a plaintiffs' attorney, winning more than a billion dollars in his three largest verdicts—a 1986 case against Monsanto, a 1988 case against Tenneco, and (after Johnson) a 1993 case against Amoco[9]— this was his first breast implant case and he clearly intended to make it good. After his stunning victory, his firm overnight became the vortex of breast implant litigation, with some 700 cases pending by the end of 1992.[10]

Plaintiffs' attorneys like to present themselves as the champions of the little people, and some of them are. But many of them are far from being little people themselves. John O'Quinn, for example, was listed in a 1989 *Forbes* magazine article as the eighth highest paid trial lawyer in the United States, with a gross income of $8 million in 1988. (Of the top ten, six were from Texas, five from Houston.) In 1989, according to *Forbes*, he was expected to make over $50 million, because of the breach-of-contract verdict against Tenneco.[11] With his explosive entry into breast implant litigation in the Pamela Johnson case, his fortunes improved. By mid-1995 his firm had 2,000 clients with breast implants, very few of whom intended to take part in the class-action settlement.[12] *Forbes* featured O'Quinn again in a July 1995 issue, referring to him as the "king of torts." O'Quinn told *Forbes* that his average verdict in a breast implant case is $10 million (yes, that would be $20 billion if all of his 2,000 clients went to court).[13] This prospect is a powerful incentive for the implant manufacturers to do business with O'Quinn and settle out of court. According to his partner, by mid-1995 the firm had settled 200 cases for over $1 million each and another 300 for less than that. About 70 percent of the firm's cases are referred to it by other lawyers, who receive a portion of the fee.[14] This consolidation of Houston cases in the hands of O'Quinn, Kerensky, McAninch, and Laminack increases the firm's considerable clout with the manufacturers. It is impossible to say exactly how much in fees the firm's 2,000-some clients with breast implants will generate for it, but its average out-of-court settlement is now rumored to be about a million dollars.[15] One can only imagine how the name "O'Quinn" is greeted within the walls of Bristol-Myers Squibb and Dow Corning.

There is no doubt that John O'Quinn stands out in a city full of vivid, swashbuckling characters. According to *Fortune* magazine, he is now worth about half a billion dollars.[16] Not that his demeanor is aggressive or combative. Far from it. At fifty-three, O'Quinn is big and imposing, but his manner in the courtroom is soft-spoken and deliberate. He talks to the jury in a direct, down-home manner, and treats the plaintiff with courtly solicitude. In the breast implant cases, he appears as the compassionate protector of helpless women, a formula that probably goes over better in Houston than it would in New York. Like Kossovsky, O'Quinn is very careful not to overtax the jurors' minds. He told the *National Law Journal* that he always begins with "a five-minute explanation that is so simple a 12-year-old child could understand."[17] His easy manner, however, cloaks an implacable will to win, undeniable shrewdness in knowing just how to do it, and the cockiness that comes with doing it so often.

O'Quinn is simply an extreme example of the way in which many plaintiffs' attorneys have benefited from the breast implant controversy. For every successful verdict or out-of-court settlement, a plaintiffs' lawyer receives a contingency fee of roughly a third. Dow Corning has estimated that cases that go to court cost them on average a million dollars (less than O'Quinn's firm gets, but not bad). Although manufacturers refuse to disclose the average amount of out-of-court settlements, they cannot be trivial or women would not accept them. For a lawyer with many cases, then, the fees add up rapidly. When Judge Sam Pointer stipulated that a billion of the $4.25 billion class-action settlement would go to the lawyers involved, it seemed that he was handing them a windfall. In reality, he was curbing them by limiting them to a 25 percent contingency fee, considerably lower than they are accustomed to.

PLAINTIFFS' ATTORNEYS in breast implant cases who were not involved in the class settlement had two clear interests: first, that women opt out of the settlement to make individual claims, and second, that scientific evidence not emerge to undermine the premise that breast implants cause disease. Women were initially given a deadline of June 17, 1994, to opt out of the settlement. By coincidence, that was one day after the Mayo Clinic study was published in the *New England Journal of Medicine.* The *Journal* was as usual available to the media a few days before the publication date, with the understanding that news releases would be delayed until publication. In the same issue was my editorial commenting on the disjunction between the courtroom activity and the scientific findings. Almost immediately I received phone calls from reporters who had spoken with plaintiffs' attorneys eager to discredit the Mayo Clinic, the *New England Journal of Medicine,* and me personally. They pointed out that the Mayo Clinic research was partially funded by the American Society of Plastic and Reconstructive Surgeons' Educational Foundation, which in turn received funds from Dow Corning and other breast implant manufacturers. According to the plaintiffs' attorneys, this automatically disqualified the study from serious consideration.

A few plaintiffs' attorneys went so far as to imply that I had for some reason colluded with the implant manufacturers to delay publication of the Mayo Clinic study until precisely the opt-out week.[18] The ostensible purpose was to dissuade women from opting out of the class-action settlement and hiring their own attorneys. According to this reasoning, if there was evidence casting doubt on a link between implants and connective tissue disease, women might not do as well in court as they expected. They might decide it was better just to stay in the class settlement. When I first heard this accusation, I was puzzled. Assuming for the moment I was captive to the breast implant manufacturers, why would I wait until the last minute to publish the Mayo Clinic study? Wouldn't I want to publish it as soon as possible so that even fewer women would opt out? The answer, according to reporters who had spoken with plaintiffs' attorneys, was that by waiting I would sow confusion in the minds of undecided women, but do so when they no longer had time to check with their attorneys (who presumably would have straightened them out by assuring them the Mayo Clinic study was invalid). Aside from the irrationality of the theory, it ignored the fact that Dr. Sherine Gabriel, first author of the study, had already presented her findings at a meeting the previous fall.[19] It also overlooked the fact that the alleged plot would have required the collusion of the other editors at the *New England Journal of Medicine,* including the editor-in-chief. What was clear was that the plaintiffs' attorneys wanted to blame the messenger (the *New England Journal of Medicine*) for the message (the results of the Mayo Clinic study).

In fact, the Mayo Clinic study was accepted and scheduled in the usual way on April 14, about two months before the publication date. Dow Corning had indeed been a contributor to the educational arm of the American Society of Plastic and Reconstructive Surgeons, which had in turn awarded a grant to the Mayo Clinic for the breast implant study. The grant from the plastic surgeons was only a part of the funding of the study, most of which came from the NIH and the Mayo Clinic itself. The source of funding for the study was duly disclosed in the *Journal,* as is our general practice, but not the fact that Dow Corning had contributed to it. However, the terms of the grant precluded any influence of Dow Corning on the study. The grant, which I was later assured was awarded after the study was designed and launched, was accepted by the Mayo Clinic on condition that the plastic surgeons' Educational Foundation (and, of course, Dow Corning) would not have access to the results until after the study was completed. They would also have no control over whether or where the study was published. (This is standard practice when a reputable research institution receives a grant from industry.) The plaintiffs' attorneys, however, despite their own obvious financial interest in the matter, insisted that the grant from the plastic surgeons invalidated the study.

When the paper was scheduled for publication, neither I nor any of the other editors had yet heard about the class-action settlement, let alone the opt-out provision. We did, however, realize that the study would receive a good deal of public attention. Anticipating this, we faxed the authors a query: because of the intense concern about breast implants, did they wish to disseminate their findings immediately to the media? We thus made an exception to our usual policy of asking authors not to discuss their work with reporters until the full report is published. Dr. Gabriel, the senior author of the study, immediately responded that she preferred to wait until the publication date. So much for the theory that the editors had kept the study quiet to cause last-minute panic.

Some plaintiffs' attorneys were not satisfied. In October 1994, I was called from a meeting in the editorial offices of the *Journal* and handed a subpoena that originated with a Houston plaintiffs' attorney. It demanded that I produce a large number of documents, most of which do not exist. In addition to all records of the peer review of Gabriel's study, I was to hand over any documents that showed that breast implant manufacturers paid me to publish the Mayo Clinic study. For example, I was to produce "all documents reflecting or relating to any payments made by any of the above listed entities [several manufacturers of breast implants and their parent companies were named above] to deponent or the *New England Journal of Medicine* concerning the Mayo Clinic study of Dr. Sherine E. Gabriel." There were no such payments, and therefore no documents reflecting or relating to them. The Massachusetts Medical Society, owners of the *New England Journal of Medicine,* filed a motion to quash the subpoena, which was successful. Our attorneys pointed out that the subpoena constituted a blatant fishing expedition. Nevertheless, in April 1995, I received another subpoena from the same attorney. Again, the Massachusetts Medical Society filed a motion to quash, which again was successful.

I was not the only one to be handed subpoenas originating in Texas. Gabriel herself was subpoenaed, as were other epidemiologists working in the field. As mentioned in Chapter 1, they were asked to produce absurdly large volumes of documents, many of no conceivable relevance. The harassment took its toll. Gabriel described her ordeal in a May 16, 1995, *New York Times* article.[20] According to the report, plaintiffs' attorneys in Houston have demanded that she produce "over 800 manuscripts from researchers that were here, they want hundreds of data bases, dozens of file cabinets and the entire medical records of all Olmsted County women, whether or not they were in the study." Gabriel found the burden of these demands staggering. Dealing with them has taken an enormous amount of her time and energy and compromised her ability to do her work. In her view, her experience and that of others will have a chilling effect on implant research. No one will want to do it, given the likely consequences. Even more important, this use of subpoena powers threatens the very existence of several large epidemiologic databases, including the one at the Mayo Clinic. These databases depend on the cooperation of large numbers of individual doctors. If doctors believe that their patients' records cannot be kept private because they might be subpoenaed, they will simply pull out.

WHAT IS GOING ON IN TEXAS? Readers will wonder why so much of the breast implant shenanigans seem to be centered there. Of the nearly 8,000 American women who opted out of the class-action settlement, most are from Texas.[21] Why is that? And why do the plaintiffs' attorneys do so well there? A convergence of factors makes for a fascinating story of justice, Texas style. First, Texas is one of a minority of states that elects all its state judges, including members of the state supreme court. There are no limits on the amount an individual may contribute to these political contests.[22] Plaintiffs' attorneys give handsomely and it is hard to believe that they do this for purely altruistic motives.

Texas also demonstrates a casual attitude toward the solicitation of clients by attorneys. Texas plaintiffs' attorneys solicit women with breast implants openly and aggressively.[23] (They are now launched on a similar campaign to find women with Norplant contraceptive implants.[24]) When women answer these solicitations, which virtually promise free money, plaintiffs' attorneys work with certain doctors to build a case.[25] In 1989, John O'Quinn apparently attracted attention even in Texas for his methods. According to *Forbes* and other published sources, he was brought before the bar for violating professional standards involving solicitation and fee splitting. (This was before he got into breast implant litigation.) He received a public reprimand and agreed to perform 100 hours of community service and pay a fine of $38,000.[26]

To me, as a physician, the most sobering aspect of breast implant litigation in Texas is the collaboration between a small group of doctors and plaintiffs' attorneys. This is by no means unique to Texas, but it seems to have reached its most extreme forms there. Plaintiffs' attorneys send potential clients to certain doctors, whose practices may consist largely of such patients and who may be paid directly by the attorneys. The arrangement is problematic at best. It is all the more worrisome in view of the fact that the diseases sought are so ill-defined.[27]

Dr. Robert I. Lewy, a Houston hematologist, is an example of a doctor whose work is now largely devoted to women with breast implants who are considering litigation. He set up a foundation called Breast Implant Research, Inc. The foundation's brochure suggests, without explicitly saying so, that autoimmune disease may be inevitable in women with breast implants.[28] He hastens to add that the disorder is unlikely to conform to the usual diagnostic criteria, in part because it has components of both connective tissue disease and multiple sclerosis. Lewy employs a large battery of tests for diagnosis, including an MRI of the brain and a bone scan, some of them very expensive. Despite the length of the list, the fact remains that there is no specific test or group of tests that is known to diagnose silicone-related illness.

If women are not alarmed for themselves by the dire predictions in Lewy's brochure, they must surely be frightened for their children. The brochure alleges that children of mothers with implants may have "scleroderma problems of the esophagus causing swallowing difficulties in children who were nursed, though we see similar problems in those not nursed." It goes on to say, "We test children the same way we test mothers, and often, even if there are no symptoms, they have similar results at times almost as if they have implants themselves with antibodies to silicone or lupus or brain masses." This is scary stuff. (Remember, the class-action settlement provides for claims by children of women with implants.)

Lewy implies that breast implants should be removed ("The more we know about silicone, the less we want to be anywhere near it!"). He also recommends repeat tests every three months or oftener for women who are taking a variety of medications. (Lewy points out, however, that women can still have autoimmune disease even with normal tests and no symptoms.) He promises a complete report of the test results, contained in a letter addressed to the person who referred the woman. The diagnosis, he says, may be in "conventional medical terms ('lupus,' etc.)," despite the fact that it may not be strictly accurate. Lewy suggests that the clinical evaluation could be done by another doctor using a form supplied by Lewy. (The woman is instructed to reassure the second doctor that he or she will not be called on to testify.) The second doctor simply needs to document the relevant symptoms (and they are listed in detail for both client and doctor). As Lewy candidly explains in the brochure, "the manufacturers (and frankly, jurors) value a woman's case much lower who claims that lots of things are wrong with her, but who has never complained of these problems to a doctor or sought treatment, than a claim that has outside documentation of the complaints. Documentation of the complaint by medical personnel is important, but *diagnosis of a condition related to them* (such as chronic fatigue, myalgia, fibromyalgia, scleroderma, nerve abnormalities) *is of great value to your claim"* (Lewy's italics). Lewy apparently does not hold out much hope that women with breast implants may be healthy. According to the *New York Times,* 93 percent of the implant recipients he has seen were diagnosed as ill. Over 90 percent were referred to him by lawyers—who, of course, receive the results and diagnosis. Lewy's income in 1994 was $2 million.[29]

At least one woman, a nurse, was apparently frightened enough by Lewy to seek a second opinion. She later told her story to reporter John Getter on KHOU, a Houston CBS affiliate. Identified only as "Marsha" and filmed in shadow, the nurse said she did not think she was ill or had connective tissue disease. She visited a plaintiffs' attorney merely to find out what she might be entitled to under the class-action settlement. The attorney sent her to Lewy. Although she said she did not actually see Lewy, a large number of tests were performed, including an MRI, which she was instructed to have at a particular facility across town, not at her own hospital. After the tests, she was told she had a lupus-like disease, and was given a letter to that effect addressed to the attorney who had referred her. The nurse was genuinely alarmed to hear that she had what she knew was a serious disease. She was particularly concerned because she was told she should be treated with corticosteroids, which she knew could cause damaging side effects.[30] Frightened, she went to see her longtime physician, Dr. David Pate, who could find no evidence of illness. When I spoke with Pate, he said that he assumed the diagnosis was based on a borderline antinuclear antibody test (which is not uncommon in normal people) and an MRI that was reported as "abnormal." Marsha told her doctor that her conscience would not let her go ahead with the virtual invitation to sue or make a claim under the class settlement. But in her interview with Getter, she added "my family will kill me." Getter asked whether they had wanted her to "take the money and run." Marsha replied, "I think so."

Lewy is not the only doctor in Texas to make a good living from women with breast implants. Houston neurologist Dr. Bernard Patten was featured in a 1994 "CNN Presents" program on breast implants called *Fire and Fury*, Part 4: "The Merchants of Fear."[31] Judy Woodruff, in her introduction to the program, said, "In the medical debate over the dangers of breast implants it is easy for women to fall prey to panic and to grasp at any hope for help. Are there medical hucksters out there cashing in on that panic for personal profit?" Answering the question, correspondent Kathy Slobogin spoke of "a thriving cottage industry of doctors, labs and treatment centers selling dubious science, pushing questionable diagnoses and treatments." Patten performed nerve biopsies on women with breast implants, and, according to CNN, contended that 80 percent of these women had nerve damage. Colleagues at Baylor College of Medicine, where Patten was on the faculty (he has since retired), examined some of the biopsy specimens at CNN's request and could find no such damage, nor had other neurologists seen the phenomenon. This did not stop

Patten from prescribing risky and expensive treatments. One woman interviewed on CNN said that her treatments, which included intravenous gamma globulin, corticosteroids, and antimetabolites, cost about $10,000 a month. Her three hospitalizations cost $30,000 each. She said that she did not feel any better, but that Patten told her that without the treatments, "You'll be very surprised how quickly you will go downhill, and you could potentially die." According to CNN, Patten admitted in legal depositions to making more than $300,000 a year from his breast implant patients.

And what of the scientific experts, those who testify in court or, more often, consult for attorneys? There are paid witnesses and consultants on both sides. Some of them undoubtedly involve themselves because they have strong feelings about the merits of the case. But the money is not bad. *Medical-Legal Aspects of Breast Implants,* a newsletter published by Leader Publications, reports in its April 1995 issue that the going rate for plaintiffs' experts is $300 to $600 per hour. (The board of editors of this newsletter, which costs a hefty $155 for 12 issues, includes a number of plaintiffs' attorneys, as well as Norman Anderson and Sybil Goldrich of Command Trust Network.) In the same story, the newsletter reports that one doctor who specializes in filling out paperwork said he charges about $950 for a consultation and dealing with the forms. He estimates that he has earned about a million dollars doing this.[32]

Nir Kossovsky, who testified in the Hopkins and Johnson cases, developed a blood test for silicone-related disease, called Detecsil Anti-SSAA(x) Test Battery. The test was performed by SBI Laboratories in Pittsburgh, a company founded for the purpose by Kossovsky, along with his wife and father.[33] All that is required for the test is a sample of blood and $350. SBI promoted Detecsil (the name is a contraction of the words "detect silicone") as providing "a definitive answer to whether subjects are experiencing an immune response to silicone." This promotional material, which appeared in lawyers' magazines, got SBI in trouble with the FDA, because it suggested the test could diagnose silicone-related illness (if it exists). In fact, there is no test that can do this. Kossovsky, according to CNN, received two FDA warning letters stating that his company had misbranded the test and was in violation of federal regulations.[34] Interestingly, the Dow Corning secret documents reveal that in 1982, when Kossovsky was a medical student, his adviser asked the company to fund Kossovsky while he conducted a study of implants. He was turned down. Since then, Kossovsky has been a key figure in promulgating the theory that implants cause disease.

To a remarkable extent, the breast implant story is about greed and its consequences—particularly the opportunism of plaintiffs' attorneys and their medical associates. But what about the plaintiffs themselves? Are they venal or are they innocent victims? This is perhaps the most vexing of the issues in this story. The answer is undoubtedly different for different women. Some of them, like Mariann Hopkins, are indeed seriously ill. They have heard that breast implants cause disease, and they cannot be blamed for accepting that proposition. After all, in their minds, they are living proof of it. To them, the implant manufacturers are clearly guilty of selling dangerous devices, perhaps knowingly, and the companies should be made to pay for it. Many more women with implants are not seriously ill. But because they are already convinced that implants cause disease, they immediately attribute ordinary symptoms of life, such as fatigue, muscle aches, or insomnia, to the devices. To them, even minor symptoms take on ominous meaning as portents of serious disease. And their conviction that they are at risk probably magnifies their symptoms. When people are afraid that they might have a serious disease, they often feel worse than they would if they had no such concerns. A third group of women feel fine, but because of the publicity, they are concerned that they might become sick in the future. About half the women who registered for the class-action settlement fall into this category. Finally, among all large groups of people are some opportunists. There is no reason to believe that women with breast implants are any different in this respect. The opportunists among them see that easy money is available and they decide to reach for some of it. Women like the nurse who was sent to see Lewy (and was dismayed by the gravity of Lewy's diagnosis) can be powerfully tempted by the situation. Although she resisted the temptation, it is unlikely that all such women do. Women with breast implants are just as diverse as any other large population, and there is no reason to believe that they are all the same—either in their health or in their character. But it can be very difficult to distinguish the ill from the worried well and from the opportunists. What is certain is the widespread and genuine alarm. The next chapter considers why the public is so ready to embrace stories of health hazards.

8

AMERICANS AND HEALTH NEWS: THE ALARM OF THE DAY

There seems to be some sort of planned obsolescence now to medical news.

—Ellen Goodman,
April 17, 1994

The breast implant story was, I believe, all but inevitable, given the social context in which it unfolded. Its shape conformed almost exactly to a number of important features in contemporary American society. One feature is the way the media convey health news. Television, radio, newspapers, and magazines were eager to trumpet the dangers of breast implants. Danger is a story; safety is not. With the extraordinary growth in media outlets, reporters must compete ever more desperately for stories. All important news tends to be rapidly exhausted by blanket coverage on all sides. Reporters who still have time and space to fill are then reduced to spinning out and inflating increasingly trivial details and ever more baseless speculation (witness the exhaustive, often tedious coverage of the O. J. Simpson trial). Health news, like celebrity murders or political sex scandals, is a particularly rich lode to mine, because the interest is already there—it doesn't have to be drummed up. Everyone would like to live a long, healthy life, and everyone wants to avoid health hazards. Thus, the media compete particularly avidly for stories about medical risks. Turn on any network morning television show or pick up any newspaper, and there is almost certain to be a story about some new peril to our health. The march of stories is remarkably rapid and fickle. Today's hazard tends to obliterate yesterday's. The fear that asbestos insulation causes lung cancer yields to the fear that exposure to lead causes mental retardation, which in turn gives way to concern that electromagnetic fields from household appliances and power lines generate leukemia and brain cancer. It is, after all, difficult to worry about everything at once. Concern that Agent Orange, used as a defoliant in Vietnam, caused a variety of illnesses gave way to worries that veterans of the Gulf War are suffering from their own mysterious malady. And so on: Alar on apples, radon in the basement, alcohol, estrogen, cigarette smoke, and hot dogs—all said to cause cancer. Pregnant women are particularly vulnerable to the anxieties generated by medical news stories. The list of cautions for them is virtually endless.

The price of this barrage is that we begin to feel we live in a sea of toxins and dangerous habits. The sense of peril is exacerbated by the fact that we know full well we are increasingly dependent in our daily lives on technology and the science that generates it. Naturally, the more curious among us wonder what all this technology is doing to us. Should we worry about electromagnetic fields, sick buildings, insecticides, food additives, lead, and asbestos? Are they destroying our health without our even knowing it? As the media incessantly discover and inflate new threats, many of us feel increasingly vulnerable to unseen dangers we don't understand. Unfortunately, too many Americans react with an odd mix of cynicism and gullibility, stemming from an increasingly distrustful view of the world.

Distrust as a worldview is not hard to understand in a society as complex as ours, particularly when there are indeed all sorts of things "out there" that can harm us. Difficult times add to the paranoid view. When people are worried about losing their jobs or maintaining their standard of living, when they are concerned about crime and social unrest, when they see greed and corruption all around them, they come to distrust nearly everything. This includes big government and big business—the institutions that should be making our lives better but seem always to be making them worse. Thus, if we hear that asbestos insulation is causing a plague of lung cancer, it must be true and it must be because rapacious businesses don't care and corrupt government is covering for them. In the case of breast implants, there is no doubt that there was a predilection to believe that the breast implant manufacturers had knowingly marketed dangerous devices and that the FDA had let them get away with it for years.

Citizens' advocacy groups, while in many cases performing great service, have tended to feed the paranoia. When Ralph Nader first began his consumer crusades, he provided a useful antidote to the mythology that business somehow "cares" about its customers. Nader and other consumer advocates supplied a dose of reality: business cares primarily about its market share, not the welfare of its customers. To be sure, manufacturers cannot be too obviously cavalier about matters of safety or they will lose their customers, but they have little reason not to try to get away with as much as possible. But as the consumer movement itself became a sort of industry, the method of carefully collecting evidence of wrongdoing, then exposing it, gave way to a fusillade approach. Never mind the evidence, everyone who might be doing wrong probably is. If Dow Corning is competing with McGhan to sell as many breast implants as possible and doesn't bother to establish their safety, then it is tempting to leap to the conclusion that implants probably *aren't* safe. And from there, it's another easy jump to assuming that they are very dangerous, and that the manufacturers knew that all along. I suspect that these kinds of leaps in logic led Sidney Wolfe, the director of Nader's Health Research Group, to assume the worst and act on that basis.[1]

If Americans responded to medical news stories more critically, we would not be as vulnerable as we are to recurrent, often baseless health scares. How should we respond? With a large dose of skepticism—which is not the same as cynicism. If, for example, there is a report that some food or habit or device is dangerous, people should ask themselves whether the news comes from a usually reliable source, whether it comes from one source or many, whether the alleged danger is large or small, and whether it is consistent with everything else we know about the subject. Then, unless the evidence is overwhelming or the problem urgent, we should defer a final judgment. The information can be stored away on a mental shelf until further information is forthcoming. Not all Americans are knowledgeable enough to perform such a preliminary analysis, at least not in all cases, but in my view most could do much better than they do. Why don't they?

One possible reason lies in the entertainment value of scientific scares. Recent books (*The Hot Zone,* for example) and movies (*Outbreak*) about runaway viruses are ample evidence of this, adding variations on the venerable Frankenstein staples. As the line between fiction and nonfiction is increasingly blurred in the media, news of medical dangers takes on some of this entertainment value. Reports that cellular phones may cause brain cancer or that the nearby nuclear power plant is unsafe intrigue us and give us lively topics for conversations with friends. Recall that Connie Chung was the person who alerted us to the putative dangers of breast implants and the conspiracy to hide them. Her forum was one of an increasingly popular genre of television magazine shows that are hybrids of entertainment and news. Yes, we really do want to learn what will keep us healthy and what is a threat to our lives, but that is not the only motivation in embracing news of health risks. We also want to be entertained. Charges of a conspiracy by big business to unleash dangerous products on the public, often with the alleged complicity of government agencies, add to the inherent interest of the story and therefore to its entertainment value. Righteous indignation is a strong stimulant and it can be a tight social bond among like-minded people.

Cynicism is much easier than skepticism, because it requires no distinctions. We needn't distinguish between reliable evidence and unreliable evidence, between big dangers and small ones, between likely effects and unlikely ones, between the reasonable and the bizarre. Yielding to cynicism over skepticism is therefore an easy way out. It also dovetails with our increasingly paranoid interpretation of all sorts of events.[2] Blanket cynicism gives the illusion of understanding and even certainty in an increasingly unpredictable world. It offers a consistent worldview. Any health scare can be interpreted by the cynic as the "establishment" once more neglecting the interests of the public in favor of big business or some other elite. There are no uncertainties. In addition, if we are cynical enough, we don't have to think too much about the substance of each health scare. Being absolved from thinking about science can be a great relief to people who find the prospect daunting. Many people willingly abandon whatever scientific skepticism they might muster in favor of political cynicism.

But the opposite side of the coin of cynicism is gullibility. If there are no distinctions to be made, then everything is equally likely. Imagining white cells gobbling up malignant cells is as likely to cure cancer as surgery. So are coffee enemas and macrobiotic diets. Acupuncturists, herbalists, and homeopaths are as effective in treating heart disease as cardiologists. And new diseases that are impossible to define are accepted wholesale every generation, with very little evidence, usually to account for fatigue and malaise—inevitable accompaniments of human existence since the beginning of time. Early in this century these symptoms were attributed to something called neurasthenia. Later, chronic mononucleosis was the favored diagnosis, until it was supplanted by chronic fatigue syndrome. More recently, a group of self-styled experts known as clinical ecologists have introduced the diagnosis of total body allergy or total chemical sensitivity for the same sort of nonspecific complaints. Each incarnation has been embraced by a large section of the public, who prefer the modish diagnosis to interpreting the symptoms as overwork or depression—or simply chalking them up to an unknown disorder.

Cynicism and gullibility together produce a penchant for magical thinking and the suspension of logic. Cynicism produces disdain for the traditional methods and sources of information; gullibility leads us to embrace idiosyncratic ones instead. Charlatans and opportunists have been quick to take advantage of these traits. Bookstores are filled with self-help books that imply that sickness and death are optional or character flaws. Their authors tell us that we can overcome even the most deadly diseases. If readers will only follow the author's regimen, which usually has to do with exercising the authority of the mind over the body, they are assured of a long, healthy life. Some authors, of course, proudly claim that their regimens are resisted or suppressed by the "medical establishment," thereby tapping into the cynicism that is so important in promoting these books. In addition, of course, the whole notion that each of us can somehow ward off disease and death more or less indefinitely is enormously appealing to our wish for more control in our lives.[3]

The breast implant story contains all the elements guaranteed to generate public ferment and misunderstanding. Big business is accused of selling a dangerous product to its customers and covering up proof of the danger. The FDA inexplicably sits on its hands for 16 years. The diseases caused by implants are deadly, but very subtle. There is no sure test for them. The disorders may be different from classic connective tissue disease, but then again they may not be. Only certain people can diagnose the diseases for sure. The medical profession is suppressing the truth, but gallant individuals—plaintiffs' attorneys, consumer advocates, and a few maverick scientists—are forcing it out. Adding to the mix is a strong anti-science mood among many Americans.[4] Perhaps the mood is a reaction to the exalted intellectual status scientists enjoyed for several decades after World War II. Whatever the reason, a growing number of Americans view scientists as just one more group of elitists and the scientific establishment as no more to be trusted than any other establishment. This view is particularly pronounced among a small segment of the feminist movement.

Given all the social forces at work in the breast implant controversy—the desperate competition within the media for a story, the reciprocal desire of the audience for entertainment, the cynicism and gullibility of the public about science, the widespread tendency toward paranoid interpretations of events, and the anti-scientific position of many Americans—it is perhaps not so surprising that most Americans believe that breast implants cause terrible diseases, despite the lack of any evidence that they do. In the next chapter, I will discuss the ambivalent view of the American public toward science and the consequences of this ambivalence. In the remainder of this chapter I will consider in more detail the public response to news of health risks and why it is sometimes so at odds with the scientific view.

IN CHAPTER 5, I described epidemiologic studies as the scientific method by which we can learn about risk factors in our lives. Habits of daily life are becoming increasingly important in epidemiologic research for several reasons. First, the most important causes of illness and death in the United States are chronic diseases of unknown cause, such as coronary heart disease and cancer. No longer do Americans get sick or die predominantly from infections, for which the causes are usually well known. Until the early twentieth century, infectious diseases were still major scourges, but with the introduction of good sanitation and a vast armamentarium of antimicrobial drugs, that changed. Since then, the life expectancy of Americans has nearly doubled, and we are now living long enough to develop a whole host of chronic diseases that come with age, such as hardening of the arteries, cancer, and arthritis. By and large, the causes of these diseases remain mysterious, but there is a good deal of evidence that most of them have multiple, not single, causes. Each contributing cause is therefore a risk factor, not the sole cause. Eliminating one risk factor

may lower the chances of getting the disease, but not eliminate the risk altogether. There is plenty of evidence that many
chronic diseases are influenced by environmental as well as genetic factors. For example, heart disease is far more common
in the United States than it is in Japan. At first glance, this fact
may seem to suggest a genetic cause. But Hawaiians of Japanese descent have a risk intermediate between that of the
Japanese and that of white Americans. Furthermore, the risk
in the United States is declining at a rate too fast to ascribe to
genetic changes.[5] The inescapable conclusion is that there
are features of the two cultures—not genes—that underlie
much of the differences in incidence. Clearly, the way we live
and the things we eat, drink, and breathe matter.

Americans want very much to know what the risk factors
are for heart disease and cancer and Alzheimer's disease and
birth defects, and all the other more or less mysterious diseases that threaten our health. We are particularly avid for
news of medical research that focuses on diet and lifestyle.
After all, we can do something about that. If something we
eat or do is a threat or a benefit, we want to know so that we
can change our lives accordingly. This emphasis has become
so extreme that for many Americans good health is largely a
matter of living right. No one gets sick anymore just because
of bad luck or factors beyond our control. Instead, we feel we
can ward off many if not most diseases and illnesses simply by
knowing what foods to eat, what supplements to consume,
and what leisure activities to pursue. This belief is fed by the
new emphasis on preventive medicine as a solution to rising
costs in health care. We are responsible for our own health.
Millions now eat low-fat, high-fiber diets, take antioxidant vitamin supplements, drink alcohol only in moderation, stay
slim, and exercise regularly. And in some respects the efforts

seem to be paying off. The incidence of heart disease in the United States, for example, has plummeted—particularly among the well educated—as these lifestyle changes have become more common.

But there are problems. We are getting too much advice from too many directions. No one could possibly follow it all. Furthermore, much of the advice is contradictory. One research study reaches one conclusion; another on the same subject reaches the opposite conclusion. No sooner do Americans substitute margarine for butter than it is announced that a new study shows margarine is worse.[6] After research shows that oat bran lowers cholesterol[7] and Americans are learning to like it, another study shows it doesn't work.[8] When we substitute low-calorie saccharin for high-calorie sugar, we find that one study shows saccharin causes bladder cancer,[9] but another study doesn't.[10] Some research demonstrates that beta carotene and vitamin E are good for you,[11] but other studies show that not only aren't they good for you, but they could be dangerous.[12] One study shows that electromagnetic fields are associated with an increased risk of leukemia[13]; another finds no increased risk of leukemia, but an increased risk of brain cancer.[14] Women who are grappling with the seemingly impossible task of deciding whether to take postmenopausal estrogen hear of a study that shows it increases the risk of breast cancer,[15] only to learn a few weeks later that another study shows it doesn't.[16] What is a health-conscious American supposed to believe? Sometimes the media echo the sense of frustration, or pretend to. Under the title "Diet Roulette," the *New York Times* editorialized about the margarine/butter controversy, "No wonder health-conscious Americans often feel they just can't win."[17] Columnist Ellen Goodman implied it was all a plot. "There seems to be some sort of planned obsolescence now to medical news. Today's sure cure is tomorrow's poison pellet. Fresh research has a sell-by date that is shorter than the one on the cereal box."[18] Her exasperation may have been more feigned than real, but it certainly played into the feelings of her readers.

Why the barrage of contradictory reports? Why can't medical researchers get it right the first time? The problem, in my view, has to do with the differences in the way scientists do their work and the way the media do theirs. Consider how scientists study risk factors. When researchers investigate a possible risk factor, they do an epidemiologic study to see whether the disease in question is more likely in people who are exposed to the possible risk factor than it is in those who are not. As explained in Chapter 5, the usual method is a cohort or case-control study. To review briefly, a cohort study looks at a group of people who are exposed to the possible risk and a group who are not, and follows them over time to see how many people in each group get the disease in question. A case-control study looks at a group of people who already have the disease and a group who do not, and looks back to see how many in each group were exposed to the possible risk factor under study. In either case, the important questions are whether there is a difference between the two groups, how big the difference is, and how certain we are that the difference we find in the sample groups is not due to chance or a mistake in the study design.

The difference between groups is often expressed as the ratio between the incidence of the disease in the exposed group and the incidence in the unexposed group. This ratio is expressed as a relative risk (or, in case-control studies, an odds ratio). For example, the relative risk for prostate cancer in men with a vasectomy, compared with men without a vasectomy, was found in one study to be 1.6.[19] This means that for every 10 men who don't have a vasectomy and develop cancer of the prostate, 16 men with a vasectomy will. Similarly, one of the recent studies of postmenopausal estrogen and breast cancer showed a relative risk of 1.3 for users of estrogen.[20] This means that for every 10 women who do not take estrogen and get breast cancer, 13 estrogen users will. The same result can be stated in different ways. Instead of saying a relative risk of 1.3, we could say that postmenopausal estrogen is associated with a 30 percent increase in the risk of breast cancer. Alternatively, since we already know that 3 or 4 of every 100 postmenopausal women will get breast cancer in the next 10 years, we could say that this study shows that estrogen increases that risk to 5 in 100. Or, to put it in yet another way, if you are a postmenopausal woman trying to decide whether to take estrogen, this study shows that your chances of remaining free of breast cancer for 10 years would decrease from over 96 percent to about 95 percent. I go through all these equivalent ways of expressing the same finding for a reason. As you can see, they have very different psychological impacts on the reader, even though they are saying the same thing. The issue of how to express or "frame" results of medical research is important, as I will show later.

There are many pitfalls in epidemiologic research.[21] In cohort studies, the two groups of people, who are well at the beginning of the study, may not have much motivation to disclose their exposure to the risk factor very accurately. I was recently asked to participate in a cohort study and was sent a formidable questionnaire to fill out. It asked for information about a wide variety of health habits over my entire life. Even if I had wanted to fill it out accurately, I doubt whether I could have. I chose not to enter the study, in part because the questionnaire was so daunting. I suspect that many women who did elect to respond simply filled the form out carelessly. In that case, many real associations between risk factors and disease might be missed. On the other hand, case-control studies may lead to spurious associations. Since the "cases" are already sick, they are more likely than well people to recall exposure to the possible risk factor. For example, mothers of babies with birth defects are more likely than mothers of healthy infants to recall being exposed to cigarette smoke or insecticides or hair spray or anything else they believe might explain what happened.

Probably the chief difficulty in epidemiologic studies is choosing groups of people who are alike in every way except for the exposure in question (in cohort studies) or the disease in question (case-control studies). Yet this is essential. Otherwise, some other difference between the groups might account for the results and badly mislead everyone. Other differences between groups that may confuse the results are termed "confounding variables." For example, cigarette smokers are more likely to drink alcohol than are nonsmokers. So when an epidemiologic study shows a link between cigarette smoking and a disease, it is necessary to determine whether the real association is with smoking or whether it might possibly be with drinking (the confounding variable in this case). It could be the combination—or even some other factor that might be different between smokers and nonsmokers.

Although there are statistical methods for neutralizing confounding variables, they are not perfect, and they are of no use whatsoever unless the confounding variables are known and measured. For example, epidemiologic studies have shown an association between premature births and lack of prenatal care, but maybe there are confounding variables that explain the association. Maybe it has nothing to do with pre-natal care itself. For example, it could be that women who can afford prenatal care are more likely to carry babies to term be-cause such women are better nourished. Similarly, one can imagine other, unknown confounding variables in this asso-ciation, or ones, such as education, that are difficult to char-acterize. Furthermore, if a confounding variable is very im-portant compared with the risk factor being studied, attempts to control for it may easily be inadequate. If, for example, some aspect of socioeconomic status is a major confounding variable in a study of a weak association, it may be necessary to characterize socioeconomic status very precisely, and even then attempts to factor out its influence may not succeed. Similarly, it's almost impossible to study other risk factors for lung cancer in people who smoke. Cigarette smoking is so powerful a risk factor that it swamps the effects of others. Even if researchers try to control for cigarette smoking by dividing the subjects into subgroups according to the number of ciga-rettes they smoke, it may not eliminate the confounding. Any remaining differences in smoking habits between groups might still obscure the effect of the risk factor being studied.

In addition to finding out whether the relative risk of dis-ease is higher in people exposed to a possible risk factor, we also want to know the size of the effect. How much higher is the relative risk? Does the exposure increase the risk manyfold, twofold, or perhaps by only 20 percent (a relative risk of 1.2)? An important reason for being concerned about the size of the effect is that unknown factors or confounding variables that are inadequately accounted for can easily produce spurious small effects or mask real ones. It is far less likely that con-founding variables obscure large effects. Cigarette smoking can badly confound a study of smog and lung cancer, but smog cannot seriously confound a study of cigarette smoking and lung cancer. This is why weak risk factors are so much harder to be sure of than strong ones.

As discussed in Chapter 6, the question of the size of the effect is very different from that of the statistical significance of the association (usually expressed as a P value or confidence interval). The P value is a measure of the probability that the finding is due to chance, and it reflects the size of the sample studied. If a study is large enough, even a very small effect may be pretty certain, just as a large effect may be due to chance in a small study. But even a statistically significant effect may still be wrong because of confounding variables or a systematic bias, such as cases being more likely to recall exposures than controls. Statistical tests of significance cannot eliminate the effects of such errors; they only deal with the effects of chance in sampling the populations being compared.

The limitations of epidemiologic research lead to certain cautions about the results. First, no one study should be taken as the final word. Nor should several very similar studies, since the same confounding variables or unappreciated biases may affect all of them. Instead, each study should be seen as one piece in a puzzle. The more studies of different designs in different populations that show similar results, the more confident we can be of the conclusions. Epidemiologists rarely place much stock in their findings without such consistency, and they shouldn't. Second, a strong risk factor is more likely to be real than a weak one. This is because confounding variables and biases are less able to confuse the situation, either by masking a risk factor or by suggesting one that doesn't exist. But they can easily mask or falsely suggest a small risk factor. For this reason, most epidemiologists are very skeptical of a relative risk below 3.0 or 4.0 if the finding is new and unanticipated. A relative risk smaller than this requires a good deal of confirmation. If the finding is biologically plausible, a weak effect is more likely to be accepted. For example, if a study showed that patients in hospitals where nurses did not wash their hands after tending each patient were twice as likely to get infections as those in other hospitals, that would be biologically plausible. If the finding were the reverse, it would not be plausible and a relative risk of 2.0 would almost certainly be chalked up to a confounding variable or to some unsuspected bias.

I GO THROUGH these technical points for a reason. They provide a backdrop for contrasting the very different way that the media deal with epidemiologic research. The news media, by definition, report new findings, not old ones. Their purpose is not to tell the world that everything is as they thought it was yesterday, but to tell us something new. And, given the frenetic competition within the media, the more unexpected the finding, the more coverage it gets. Thus, the assertion by Pons and Fleischmann, the University of Utah chemists who announced a few years ago that they had produced nuclear fusion at room temperature (cold fusion)—a highly implausible claim—was big news.[22] On the other hand, a confirmatory finding of a scientifically plausible effect is unlikely to make the news. Furthermore, a study that finds no effect will receive almost no attention from the media, even when it is important. One of the consequences of the emphasis on both newness and positive effects is that a study that erroneously finds an effect gets more attention than ten studies that didn't. For example, about 10 years ago a study was published purporting to find an association between drinking coffee and cancer of the pancreas.[23] It received an enormous amount of publicity; the authors were on television network news, and the newspapers and newsmagazines gave the study prominent coverage.[24] Later, when it became apparent that the finding was almost certainly spurious, this news was relegated to the back pages.[25]

Reporters are reluctant to downplay their stories by adding caveats. When a study finds a weak risk, reporters are not likely to emphasize how small the risk is and therefore how likely it is to be spurious. If they do, these qualifications are usually buried near the end of the story. Caveats are simply not a winning feature of news reports. Thus, weak risks, such as moderate obesity or eating red meat, may receive the same emphasis as strong risks, such as cigarette smoking or heavy drinking, and the public may react equally strongly to both. Furthermore, media reports are also likely to frame risks in the most impressive way. For example, a recent study, called the GUSTO trial,[26] compared two anti-clotting agents in the treatment of heart attacks—one agent was t-PA, the other streptokinase. At the end of the trial, 6.3 percent of the patients receiving t-PA had died, compared with 7.3 percent of the patients receiving streptokinase. This one percentage point improvement was hardly a great difference. In fact, stated another way, the study showed that the chances of surviving a heart attack increased from 92.7 percent with streptokinase to 93.7 percent with t-PA—pretty good odds with either drug. Equally accurate would be the statement that t-PA was associated with a 14 percent reduced mortality. Somehow, framed this way, the finding sounds much more impressive. And that's exactly how the media tended to frame it. Even when reporters caution their readers not to embrace too enthusiastically news of a weak effect from a single study, the headline writers may have other ideas. In the *Boston Globe,* the t-PA finding was reported under the headline "Anti-Clotting Therapy Found to

Spare Lives."[27] While technically true, the effect of t-PA was meaningful only when applied to a large population. For an individual patient, the drug offered only a trivial increase in the odds of survival.

All of this is not to say that the media are not doing their job. They are. It's just that the job is not what we might think it is. The job of reporters is to tell the public what happened, and to do so in as engaging a way as possible. In medical reporting, this means telling the audience, as dramatically as possible, what researchers did and what they concluded. Reporters do not usually include in the scope of their job providing a context—that is, analyzing the strengths and weaknesses of a whole body of scientific evidence. Nor does the job include coming up with a reasoned conclusion for the public, although good reporters often do this. Instead, most reporters simply inform the public, study by study, of whatever research is most newsworthy that day—that is, most startling.

But startling research is more likely to be wrong than confirmatory research. Solid conclusions are usually reached bit by bit. The more studies done of a particular question, the more accurate they are likely to be, as the errors of earlier studies are avoided. News of the entire sequence is unlikely to make it to the media, at least not toward its end, when it is most reliable. To be sure, the media often present very good feature stories about medical subjects. In these, reporters analyze at some length what is known about the field, what questions remain to be answered, and what the implications are. These longer, more analytic stories often appear in newsmagazines, in the health sections of large newspapers, or in the Sunday feature pages. They emphasize a body of research, not just a single study. But the lion's share of media coverage of medical research is news of a single, dramatic study, and this is where the problems lie.

One frequent justification for the media making much of weak risk factors is that they are important for the public health, if not for individuals. An individual may not see much difference between his or her chances of surviving a heart attack with t-PA or streptokinase, but for the public health, it matters. Since there are nearly 1.5 million heart attacks a year in this country, a one-percentage-point improvement in the chances of surviving translates into 15,000 lives saved. Another example: A trial using cholestyramine to lower serum cholesterol about 9 percent in middle-aged men with high cholesterol levels reduced their seven-year risk of heart attacks or sudden death from 8.6 to 7.0 percent.[28] Although such a reduction may not seem like much to an individual, particularly since it requires taking a drug with side effects, when spread over the estimated 1 million to 2 million Americans with similar cholesterol levels, it could account for up to 32,000 fewer heart attacks a year. The public health perspective has been gaining steadily in importance in the past several years, as policymakers have grown increasingly concerned about costs. Anything that reduces health-care expenditures, even if it doesn't reduce risks much for individuals, is important. But this switch in emphasis has occurred nearly subliminally. Reporters are rarely explicit about it. They may not always be aware of it themselves. Health risks continue to be reported as though they were meaningful for the individual, and, of course, people assume that the risks would not be in the news unless they were. But even well-established risk factors may have little importance for individuals. For example, the 10-year risk of death from cardiovascular disease is 4.9 percent in middle-aged men with high cholesterol levels, as compared with 1.7 percent in those with low cholesterol levels.[29] This difference in risk of about three percentage points may not be enough to induce an otherwise healthy man to try to lower his cholesterol level. Yet many American men have been led to believe that high cholesterol is a death sentence, and low cholesterol means they will have a long life.

Ellen Goodman's lament is a little different from the problems of distinguishing weak from strong risk factors, sensational from solid studies, and news of importance to individuals from news of importance to the public health. She was complaining that studies were inconsistent and often contradictory. Let's look at these complaints more closely. It is true that one study may find, say, that postmenopausal estrogen is associated with breast cancer and the next study may find that it isn't. Such inconsistency is common in medical research. It is particularly common in epidemiology, because these studies are so difficult to do. Instead of being a cause for lament, the phenomenon ought to suggest more caution in accepting the results of any one study. Caution is what inconsistency teaches scientists, and there is no reason why the public—and reporters and columnists—cannot draw the same lesson. Furthermore, the inconsistency may be more apparent than real. If a risk factor is very weak, but statistically significant, the media report this as showing an effect. Another study may have found exactly the same relative risk, but because the study was smaller, the difference was not statistically significant. The media would report the second study as showing no effect. The possibility that there was really no difference between the two study results would simply not be reported.

Goodman was also complaining about another problem. Some studies show that something is good for you in one way and bad in another. As she said, "estrogen may protect against heart disease and give you a better shot at breast cancer. If you run a lot, your bones may get brittle but your heart will stay strong. If you drink wine, you could wreck your liver but lower your bad cholesterol." There is no answer for this lament. Nature simply did not set out to make things uniformly good or uniformly bad for us. They are what they are. But the situation underscores another important problem in reporting health news. Media stories about a research study that focused on jogging and osteoporosis (Goodman's "brittle bones") too often reported the results in isolation. In reality, almost any food or activity that affects health in one way also affects it in others. It is a disservice to the public not to try to put stories about single research studies in their larger context. People feel whipsawed by science. when they are really being whipsawed by the media.

As the recent epidemiologic studies of breast implants and the diseases they are said to cause have been reported in the scientific literature, how have the media responded? By and large, very well. Since the studies have been so consistent, there has been little necessity to deal with contradictions. The limitations in the strength of the findings caused by the size of the studies have been appropriately mentioned, as were the flaws in the one study that found a link. Failure to find a difference between women with and without implants does not mean that there is no difference. The smaller the study, the more likely that a real difference will be missed. This fact is usually expressed by a "confidence interval," that is, a range of possible risks that is compatible with the evidence. In the Mayo Clinic study, for example, the relative risk for the diseases studied in women with breast implants was 1.0. This meant that compared with women without breast implants, those with implants were no more or less likely to develop the diseases in question. But because there were only 749 women with breast implants in the study, it was 95 percent possible that the relative risk was anywhere from 0.5 to 3.0. The closer to the extremes of the confidence interval, the more improbable, but it was still quite possible that breast implants were associated with as much as a threefold increase in these diseases. The press made this clear. Larger studies will have a narrower confidence interval. Therefore, the more large studies that can find no association between implants and disease, the smaller any real risk must be not to have been detected. On the other hand, if there is a risk that has been missed, larger studies are more likely to find it.

What if it turns out that there is a small risk? A quick answer would be that no risk is acceptable. In this view, if there is any risk, no matter how small, implants ought to remain banned. After all, we should accept no unnecessary threats to health. Unfortunately, the real world cannot work that way. We accept unnecessary risks to health every day. Whenever we drive our cars or take an antibiotic or eat peanut butter, we take risks. (Antibiotics, after all, can have serious side effects, peanuts contain a mold that increases the risk of liver cancer, and automobile accidents are far more important causes of death and injury than most of the health hazards that occupy our attention.) Paradoxically, then, unnecessary risks may be necessary. The important question is the size of each risk and the costs, not just in dollars, of avoiding it. If a risk is so small that it is nearly impossible to detect, then perhaps it doesn't matter, just as it might not matter to an individual whether he or she receives t-PA or streptokinase after a heart attack. Maybe we should just stop worrying and include whatever risk there is from breast implants with the multitude of small (and not so small) risks we accept willingly every day. On the other hand, we might be unwilling to accept certain small risks, but quite ready to accept others.[30] The crucial point is that we owe it to ourselves to decide these matters explicitly. Unfortunately, Americans are not very good at evaluating risks of health hazards and deciding which ones we are willing to take. Oddly enough, many of us are also reluctant to rely on science to tell us about health hazards. Increasingly, we look to other sources, and some of these sources are strange indeed. In the next chapter, I will discuss the anti-science movement that is sweeping this country and its unfortunate consequences.

9

BREAST IMPLANTS AND THE REJECTION OF SCIENCE: OTHER WAYS OF KNOWING

It's a foreboding I have—maybe ill-placed—of an America in my children's generation, or my grandchildren's generation . . . when, clutching our crystals and religiously consulting our horoscopes, our critical faculties in steep decline, unable to distinguish between what's true and what feels good, we slide, almost without noticing, into superstition and darkness.

—Carl Sagan,
1995[1]

The United States is in the midst of a groundswell of anti-science feeling. (The renewed rejection of evolution exemplifies this feeling.) It comes at a time when we are most dependent on science and the technology it generates. At first thought, it may seem paradoxical to reject science when we are most dependent on it, but perhaps it isn't. Perhaps it is human nature that the more we feel dependent on something, the more we rebel against it, much as dependent adolescents rebel against their parents. Be that as it may, the rebellion is spearheaded by a variety of groups within American society, each with its own political stance and reasons for turning against science and technology. They include humanists, multiculturalists, environmentalists, ecologists, feminists, and proponents of alternative medicine. Not all members of these groups, of course, reject science. But each movement is notable for having large contingents that do. They view science somewhat differently.

Many humanists believe that science has been oversold as the discipline with the answers. In their view, the deference to science that has characterized intellectual life for much of this century has contributed to a devaluation of humanist thought and the emergence of a callous, technology-enthralled society. In rejecting the uses to which science has been put, they also reject the scientific method and, to some extent, those who espouse it. As Paul Gross, professor of life sciences and director of the Center for Advanced Studies at the University of Virginia, and Norman Levitt, professor of mathematics at Rutgers University, point out in their book, *Higher Superstition,* rejecting science also offers academic humanists the opportunity to settle old scores.[2]

After World War II, science and scientists enjoyed a virtually unchallenged primacy in the intellectual hierarchy. Scientists, after all, were the people who were necessary to win the war, arm us for the cold war, find cures for diseases, and give us our technological creature comforts. In academia, they enjoyed the relatively lush funding that came with their usefulness. They also enjoyed great intellectual prestige. Gross and Levitt outline the implicit ranking of the various academic fields that prevailed until very recently. Academics in the "hard" sciences (physics, chemistry, biology) ranked first because they produced reliable knowledge; historians, second, because they, too, generated factual knowledge, although often tainted by speculation; economists, third, because at least their analytical methods were rigorous, even if their assumptions and sometimes their raw data were not. Next to the bottom of the hierarchy were social scientists, because they indulged in impressionistic theories dressed up in statistical costumes, and last were those in literature, because they were subjective beyond redemption. With the rejection of science, that hierarchy stands to be reversed. Humanists now speak of science as just another mode of discourse constructed by its practitioners, no more objective than any other and probably less interesting. With this reevaluation, there is no longer any reason to defer epistemologically to scientists.

Multiculturalists also have quarrels with science. To many of them, it glorifies a white, male, European construct, at the expense of the contributions of other races and cultures. And indeed, the emphasis on science and technology *is* a hallmark of Western civilization. Some multiculturalists react by disdaining science altogether. Others, however, do not reject science, but rather appropriate it, often in novel forms. Hunter Adams, for example, a proponent of Afrocentric science who was commissioned by the Portland, Oregon, public schools to design a more inclusive curriculum, accepts scientific advances, but attributes many of them to the ancient Africans. In addition, he referred to ancient Africans as "masters of magic . . . psychokinesis, remote viewing and other underdeveloped human capabilities."[3] Presumably, these are other branches of science.

The anti-science environmentalists and ecologists dislike science for its hubris. To them, the technological imperative fed by science has led to an arrogant and ultimately self-destructive assumption of dominion over nature.[4] Other groups reject science for political reasons. Many radicals, for example, see the technological fruits of science as bolstering the power of the governing classes. Technology thereby becomes one more tool of economic subjugation.[5] Moving nearer the mainstream, even good liberals are often very critical of science without rejecting it altogether. Consumer advocates such as Public Citizen's Sidney Wolfe exemplify the views of those who find the rapid progress of science as much a cause for vigilance as celebration.[6]

A particularly influential group to turn against science is a segment of the feminist movement. Feminist philosophers such as Sandra Harding, professor of philosophy at the University of Delaware, provide the intellectual framework. To them, science is inherently "androcentric," because it was largely developed by men in patriarchal societies. It is only because of the power of men that the scientific method has become universally accepted as the way to gain knowledge about the natural world. To these feminists, the scientific method would be different if it had been developed by women. Harding, for example, believes that "value-free research is a delusion," and she has compared the scientific method to "marital rape, the husband as scientist forcing nature to his wishes." She writes as though the scientific method were just one more convention that could easily be replaced by another.[7] Many feminists are receptive to this view, because they believe that the scientific method leaves out other, equally valid ways of knowing. The 1986 book *Women's Ways of Knowing* suggests that women find the scientific method uncongenial because it emphasizes logical, linear thinking at the expense of intuitive, multi-faceted thinking.[8] Of course, intuition and imagination often do play an important role in generating hypotheses in science, but logical analysis is the most useful tool, and all scientific hypotheses must ultimately stand the test of objective evidence. Some feminists do not accept these constraints, and many other women are to some extent influenced by their ideas without embracing them explicitly.

In addition to these anti-science groups, there are many individuals who react in particular against medicine and medical science. For years, the public has been ambivalent about their doctors. While most people seem to like and trust their own physicians, many believe the medical profession as a whole needs to be brought down to size. In their view, doctors for too long have been allowed to get away with insufferable arrogance. They are often not available to their patients, and when they are, they do not take the time to listen to them carefully and understand their problems. Instead, doctors either dismiss the patient altogether or rush to a high-cost technological fix. (Much of this, of course, is changing, as both doctors and patients are brought under the aegis of "managed care." Doctors will be less likely to reach for a technological fix and perhaps be less arrogant, but no less busy.) The public is also critical of medical science because it seems to promise "medical miracles" that too often aren't delivered. The media imply that medical science can do nearly anything. For example, a recent story about a substance that causes mice to lose weight appeared in one newspaper under the headline "Flabulous Discovery!"[9] The story implied that we were on the brink of a new, definitive treatment for human obesity, a highly unlikely possibility. Other media stories suggest that similar medical miracles are at hand. Many doctors feed these unrealistic expectations by being unwilling to tell patients when they do not know how to help them. Instead, they sometimes reach for one more drug or procedure, raising false hopes. Yet people still become obese, and they still get sick and die, the implied promises notwithstanding. When the public's expectations are so inflated, disillusionment is inevitable.

For women, the medical profession has presented special problems. There is no question that when medicine was an almost entirely masculine profession, women patients often were patronized. Sometimes they were the victims of what was little more than professionally sanctioned prejudice. When I was in medical school in the 1960s I was taught that dysmenorrhea was a psychiatric disorder—the physical manifestation of an attempt by women to reject the feminine role. Similarly, morning sickness was ascribed to rejection of the fetus. Patients with these problems were often treated with tranquilizers and fatherly lectures about their role in life. This sort of thing is for the most part behind us, but some of the residual outrage among women remains. Furthermore, in the view of some women, researchers have not paid enough attention to diseases that predominantly affect women, such as breast cancer and osteoporosis. That charge is debatable; what is not debatable is that the ranks of doctors and researchers have until recently consisted overwhelmingly of men.

The anti-science, anti-medicine strain in the feminist movement finds expression in the breast implant controversy. Many women see the controversy as a women's issue in a political context, as well as a biological one. Some female plaintiffs' attorneys make much of the fact that they are women championing other women in a man's world.[10] The epidemiologic studies that fail to find a connection between breast implants and disease are met with cynicism. To many feminists, scientific studies seem irrelevant and distracting in the context of a perceived widespread assault on women—first in subjecting them to implants, then in failing to respond promptly to the hazard. After all, implants are unnatural substances put in the body, and many women who have implants get sick. When scientific data are put up against their own "ways of knowing," some women ignore the science. Add to this anti-science bias the view of many women that breast implants are a manifestation of a discredited, masculine attitude that judges women primarily by their looks, and it is no wonder that some feminists believe breast implants cause disease. They *want* to believe it.

Note that the various elements of the anti-science movement have somewhat distinct grievances. Some, such as the radical environmentalists, are reacting primarily against the uses to which science is put. Others, like the academic humanists, are reacting against what they see as the exaggerated status of science. And many, like the anti-science feminists and the multiculturalists, are rejecting the scientific method.

THE ATTACK ON SCIENCE leaves a vacuum that must be filled. If science cannot provide the answers, what can? People still want to know why they are sick or unhappy, and they still want to know how the world originated and how it works. In short, while many have turned from science, people are still curious about nature and their bodies and minds. The anti-science movement inevitably carries in its wake all manner of contenders for the job of providing answers. What they have in common is a surrender, partial or complete, of reason to speculation and mysticism. But because we are people accustomed to the sound of scientific language, the surrender is often cloaked in a patois of scientific jargon.

A current example of this surrender is the apparently widespread acceptance of the proposition that large numbers of people are being abducted by aliens (who, not surprisingly, are given to a lot of sexual experimentation). The chief proponent of this proposition, Harvard psychiatrist John Mack, makes the case in a best-selling book, *Abduction: Human Encounters with Aliens.*[11] Mack, a great favorite on talk shows, gives the whole thing a scientific veneer, despite its utter lack of scientific support. He told a gathering of critics, "Other cultures have always known that there were other realities, other beings, other dimensions. There is a world of other dimensions, of other realities that can cross over into our own world."[12] All of this sounds remotely like science, particularly the part about dimensions, which is reminiscent of physics. The problem is that Mack and the other believers in alien abduction have not produced objective evidence for their proposition, which is the true hallmark of science. What we are left with, then, in the words of the philosopher Wittgenstein, is "the bewitchment of thought by language."[13]

Much of the surrender to mysticism doesn't even bother with a veneer of science. The talk shows are the forum for the most extreme examples. Once the preserve of tortured relationships and sexual idiosyncrasies, talk shows increasingly delve into the occult.[14] Psychics predict the future and reveal the identity of criminals (although seldom by name) before our very eyes. Witches explain their powers to enthralled audiences. A hypnotist on Oprah Winfrey's show described her method of marriage counseling. She simply takes the couple back through time to their past lives (called "regressing") to try to gain insight into their present problems. These are just a few of the many examples of the growing acceptance of the occult. It has an irresistible fascination for many people, perhaps because it evokes a form of magical thinking we all engaged in as children. Wish for something and it will happen. Step on a crack, break your mother's back. (If you don't want her back broken, don't step on the cracks.) Monsters are under the bed, and aliens are in the closet. As we grow older, we learn to substitute reason for magic, but the attraction of mysticism remains.

Mysticism finds its greatest appeal in healing. Sickness and death have always held terror for us, and until recently medical science itself was little more than witchcraft. Indeed, until this century, "alternative" ways of understanding disease and healing were probably more effective than orthodox medicine, since they tended to be gentler than the leeches and purges of conventional treatment. As medicine became increasingly scientific and effective, however, alternative medicine faded from the picture. Particularly after World War II, with the advent of spectacularly effective antibiotics, a number of other life-saving drugs, and safe surgery, medical science seemed to have totally eclipsed other approaches to healing.

But now, with the anti-science movement, alternative medicine is making a comeback. An article in the *New England Journal of Medicine* described the widespread use of alternative medicine in the United States in 1990.[15] It was based on telephone interviews with 1,539 randomly selected adults. The authors defined alternative or "unconventional" medicine as any mode of therapy not taught widely in American medical schools and not generally available in American hospitals. Included were relaxation techniques, chiropractic, massage, imagery, energy healing, biofeedback, hypnosis, homeopathy, and acupuncture (among others). Surprisingly, about 1 in 3 of those interviewed had used at least one unconventional therapy over the past year, and 1 in 6 had visited a provider of unconventional treatment—on average, 19 times. On the basis of their study, the authors estimated that in 1990 there were 425 million visits to providers of unconventional therapy, which exceeded the 388 million visits to primary-care physicians.

Given the widespread use of alternative medicine, it is not surprising that the establishment is taking respectful notice.

In 1992, under the prodding of Senator Tom Harkin (D-Iowa), an Office of Alternative Medicine was created at the National Institutes of Health. It is charged with studying a host of practices, such as healing by "Lakota medicine wheels," mental healing at a distance, "biofield therapeutics," and the use of shark cartilage to treat cancer, most of which would never even have engaged the attention of serious scientists a generation ago, much less the attention of the scientific establishment. Now they are taken seriously. Already in its short history, the Office of Alternative Medicine has become the center of intense controversy.[16] The dispute is fundamentally about whether the mission of the office is to evaluate alternative treatments scientifically (which would undoubtedly show many treatments to be worthless) or to take alternative treatments on their own terms and essentially document anecdotes. Obviously, the research projects funded could be expected to differ depending on which of these missions predominates. As of now, there has been no explicit resolution of the controversy, and the OAM continues in a state of uneasy ambivalence. In addition to the NIH, other bulwarks of the establishment are beginning to look at alternative medicine. One of Harvard Medical School's teaching hospitals, for example, now has a Mind-Body Medicine Institute.

Homeopathy, the school of healing based on the proposition that "like cures like," is making deep inroads on the establishment. Homeopaths believe in treating diseases with very dilute amounts of a substance that produces the same symptoms as the disease being treated. For example, if a patient has a head cold, he or she might be treated with an extremely dilute solution of onion extract (which, in larger doses, would cause a runny nose). According to the theory, the more dilute, the greater the effect—a theory that, if true, would violate most of the principles of chemistry and pharmacology. Three states—Connecticut, Nevada, and Arizona—now license homeopaths. The NIH is obligingly launching a clinical trial of the method.[17] A study, of course, is the only way to find out whether a treatment method works. Usually, however, there is some *a priori* biologic plausibility or expectation of an effect before resources are spent on a large trial. After all, not every hypothesis can be tested. But because of the popularity of many forms of alternative medicine, they will be tested anyway—and they probably should be.

In response to the anti-science movement and the growing tolerance, if not acceptance, with which it is received, some scientists are fighting back. In the summer of 1995, Gross and Levitt organized a conference of some 200 scientists, physicians, and humanists under the auspices of the New York Academy of Sciences. Called "The Flight from Science and Reason," the conference was devoted to analyzing and countering the anti-science movement. The participants discussed the paradox of people rejecting the technology on which they depend and the Western scientific tradition that created it. The most sobering aspect to many of the participants was the fact that the theoretical basis for the rejection—which some termed a romantic rebellion—comes not from religious fundamentalists, whose quarrel with science is well understood and long-standing, but from academics who regard themselves as intellectuals. Other than inspiring some op-ed pieces on the subject,[18] the conference probably did not have much effect. The horse is already out of the barn.

AND WHAT IS THE DAMAGE? Why not encourage many "ways of knowing"? What's wrong with "alternative" healing? Why not, indeed, indulge our fascination with the mystical and the occult? In my view, the disdain for science has enormous implications that reverberate far beyond the answer to any one of these questions. Throwing over science means throwing over an attachment to evidence. Viewing science as just one possible "way of knowing," amounting to little more than the customs of a white men's club, has the same result. The scientific method was not put together and then applied to questions of nature, or, as Harding would have it, forced on nature. It evolved painfully over many years, through trial and error, because it was the only method that worked. It had to be what it is. Contrary to Harding, nature forced itself on those who would study it, not the reverse. Science is the only way to reach conclusions about the physical world, including the human body. Try predicting the time and place of the next solar eclipse without it, or the sex of a baby before it is born. As Robert Park, professor of physics at the University of Maryland, said, "Science is the only means we have to sort out the truth from ideology or fraud or mere foolishness."[19] It is therefore dismaying to scientists to find that many Americans not only do not understand science, but they don't want to understand it and they don't think it's necessary that they do.

Anti-science feminism is particularly difficult for me, as a feminist, to accept. After years of women fighting for entry to the world of science, it is ironic that some of them would turn away now. Women should not permit themselves to be excluded from science, much less abandon the field. We should instead work to bring women into science at the main point of exclusion—the earliest years of grade school and even before. Girls receive strong social messages that science and math are boy subjects; English and the social sciences are girl subjects. As a woman who herself bucked this attitude (I remember being told in college that I "thought like a man" and not having enough sense to be offended by this alleged compliment), I am dismayed to see many feminists embracing the prejudice. And I am particularly appalled at the move to dismiss the scientific method itself. There are many problems with the assertion that women have their own, equally valid ways of reaching what are essentially scientific conclusions. Besides playing into the anti-feminist conceit that women can't get their little minds around scientific concepts, it caricatures the nature of science, as well as the nature of both men and women. Good scientists will attest to the role of intuition and inspiration—that is, creativity—in their work. But while such nonlinear thinking lies behind many a brilliant hypothesis, it is still necessary to test it. This requires the application of the scientific method—the dogged accumulation of evidence that will logically speak to the question. (Unfortunately, the creative revelation often turns out to be ill-conceived. In the words of Carl Sagan, "the vast majority of ideas are simply wrong."[20]) There is nothing wrong with postulating apparently unscientific hypotheses, but there *is* something wrong with failing to put them to the test. If an unconventional medical practice really works, it should be possible to demonstrate that fact. Of course, many conventional "scientific" beliefs about health and disease also are vulnerable to the same criticism of never having been tested. Some practices in medicine are based on little more than hearsay and habit. These, too, should be subjected to scientific testing.

The best reason for women not to turn against science is the same as it is for men: The scientific method works. Make no mistake, the astonishing advances in science and technology over the past couple of centuries, particularly in recent years, would have been impossible without the scientific method. Without it, we would have no immunizations, no antibiotics, no painless, safe surgery, no blood transfusions, indeed, not even clean water or electricity. We would still have a life expectancy of less than 40 years, and half our children would die before adulthood of diphtheria, measles, tetanus, and diarrhea. (Many feminists who disdain science vote with their feet on this one, taking their children to be immunized against childhood diseases even though the immunizations were developed by white men using the scientific method.) Dismissing science because it was developed by men is unwise. What needs to be done is for women to wield this powerful tool on their own behalf, not to cede the ground.

What does all this have to do with breast implants? I have discussed the anti-science movement in some detail, because it establishes the context in which the breast implant controversy developed and it greatly influences how it will unfold. When the first reports of a link between breast implants and systemic disease appeared, it was a time for skepticism. It was a time for filing away the information as unsubstantiated anecdotes, not throwing it away altogether, but certainly not giving it credence. It was a time to gather evidence. Instead, many people who heard about the reports (and the ensuing lawsuits) responded according to their political or social positions. More important, they filled the vacuum resulting from a lack of understanding about what would constitute such evidence. People could feel pretty certain about the matter based on all manner of considerations except what science had to say. Those who had dismissed the scientific method as an androcentric tool, in particular, could believe that implants caused disease because they "knew" it. To them, the anecdote was the new scientific method.

The breast implant controversy should be seen not only

in the context of the anti-science movement, but also in the context of many of the other health scares that erupt periodically. As a result of a combination of publicity, anti-science attitudes, paranoia, profiteering, and, yes, scientific evidence, a great many such scares come and go. There is sometimes little follow-up as to which ones turn out to have substance and which ones are baseless. How many Americans know that there was no evidence whatsoever that the anti-nausea drug Bendectin caused birth defects? How many know that there is no evidence for a unique syndrome that afflicts veterans of the Persian Gulf War? How many know that the hazards of asbestos and radon are probably very small except at high levels of exposure?[21] In this context, the notion that breast implants cause disease is plausible. (It is certainly a lot more plausible than alien abductions.) After all, implants are capable of doing a lot of local damage when they rupture or contractures form. The fact that the scientific evidence seems not to have affected the general view of breast implants is also not surprising, given the record on this score.

We do indeed have other "ways of knowing." They seem to satisfy all sorts of needs and wishes in our complex society, but they can't tell us whether breast implants cause disease. That question remains to be answered in the only way it can be—through science. The controversy is not over and it may not be resolved for years. In the final chapter, I will discuss the prospects for its resolution and what we can learn from this whole story.

10

WHERE WE STAND . . .
AND FOR HOW LONG

On May 15, 1995, Dow Corning filed for Chapter 11 bankruptcy protection. This is the latest, but by no means the first, example of a company brought to its knees by mass litigation. Bankruptcy protection does not mean the dissolution of the company; rather, it means that the company must be reorganized to pay its debts as ordered by the bankruptcy court. With bankruptcy, all of the claims against Dow Corning in both federal and state courts were brought under the jurisdiction of this single court. That is one advantage of bankruptcy. Instead of dealing with creditors in countless jurisdictions, the company is subject to a coherent plan crafted by one court.

Even before Dow Corning claimed bankruptcy, the class-action settlement was unraveling. Because so many women had registered, Judge Sam Pointer announced in early May that the size of the compensation for each woman would have to be reduced.[1] The original settlement included a grid showing specific amounts to be awarded to each claimant, depending on her age, the type of illness and the severity. Of the $4.25 billion, $1.2 billion was set aside for women claiming to be sick already. The remainder (minus the billion dollars for the lawyers' fees) was to cover those who became sick over the next 30 years.[2] With the registration of 440,000 women,

248,500 of whom claimed to be sick already, it was abundantly clear that the settlement, huge as it was, would not begin to cover all the claims.[3]

The number of women claiming to be sick is roughly 20 percent of all women with breast implants. I do not know the details of their claims, but if only 10 percent of them claim to have classic connective tissue disease, it would be at least double the rate in the general population. But the epidemiologic studies indicate that such a high risk is extremely unlikely. All we can say is that a very large number of women have or claim to have an unidentified illness. Ralph Knowles, of the plaintiffs' steering committee, expressed amazement at the number of claims. "There are just too many sick women," he said. "I didn't think it was going to be anything like that. If I did, we would have never agreed to the $4.25 billion."[4] Given the publicity and the extremely easy terms of the settlement, I am surprised that he was surprised. It would be natural for any woman with implants who experienced even ordinary fatigue or muscle aches to attribute her symptoms to the implants.

Regardless of whether the results should have been foreseen, it was obvious that the grid would have to be revised. Under the terms of the settlement, any such revision would require that women have an opportunity to pull out of the settlement and, if they chose, to sue individually. But if too many did, manufacturers would also pull out of the settlement, since it would no longer serve the purpose of limiting their liability. Judge Pointer, faced with the collapse of the settlement, charged the attorneys representing both sides to try to reach an accommodation—presumably involving some combination of increased contributions from the manufacturers and decreased awards for the claimants.[5] Thus, the dominoes were set to topple even before Dow Corning filed for bankruptcy.

With Dow Corning's bankruptcy, the class-action settlement fell apart, although it was not officially pronounced dead
until four months later. As the company that had sold half of
all breast implants, Dow Corning had pledged nearly half the
$4.25 billion to the settlement. Now Dow Corning was no
longer a part of it. All claims against the company would be
settled by the bankruptcy court in Michigan, its home state. It
could take years to determine which of its creditors would be
paid and how much. The remaining three companies in the
settlement—Bristol-Myers Squibb, Baxter Healthcare, and
Minnesota Mining and Manufacturing (3M)—negotiated with
the plaintiffs' steering committee throughout the long summer, but failed to reach an agreement by Judge Pointer's August 30 deadline.[6] Phone calls to Pointer's information line
(800-887-6828) were greeted with increasingly pessimistic
recorded messages. The deadline was extended. Finally, on
September 7, Judge Pointer acknowledged that the original
settlement was dead, but that the remaining three manufacturers would try to negotiate a new one.[7]

On October 2, 1995, Judge Pointer announced a new, preliminary agreement.[8] Unlike the original settlement, which applied to all women with implants made by any manufacturer,
the new terms would apply only to women with implants made
by the three participating manufacturers. Women with these
implants who claim to be sick would have three options: They
could opt out of the settlement and go it alone, they could accept a much reduced compensation based on the criteria of
the original settlement, or they could apply for higher compensation by meeting more stringent criteria for illness. Those
not claiming to be sick would be able to make claims if they
became ill in the next 15 years. Unlike the original agreement, this one would not permit compensation amounts to be
reduced or manufacturers to pull out. The costs to the man-

ufacturers were therefore open-ended, but they were estimated to be $3 billion, of which $180 million would be set
aside for the lawyers.

As this book went to press, it was not at all clear that the
new agreement would hold together any better than the old
one. Many women felt betrayed by the more stringent requirements and the lower amounts of compensation.[9] Furthermore, the agreement did not apply to about half of all
women with implants—that is, those whose implants were
manufactured by Dow Corning. But as the scientific evidence
increasingly weighed in against a connection between implants and disease, the option of suing individually seemed to
grow less promising. Thus, women who thought they had a
choice between accepting the terms of a very generous class-
action settlement or trying for a larger amount individually
found themselves with both options closing off—theoretically.
On the other hand, two developments were promising for
them. First, the federal courts and a few states decided that
Dow Corning's wealthier parent company, Dow Chemical
Company, could be held liable for the claims of women with
breast implants made by Dow Corning. In the fall of 1995, a
jury in Nevada awarded $14.1 million ($10 million of which
was punitive damages) to a woman with Dow Corning implants who sued Dow Chemical. Second, the emerging scientific evidence may have little impact. In the Nevada case, Dow
Chemical pointed to the Mayo Clinic study and the Nurses'
Health Study, but to no avail. The only certainty is that, with
the collapse of the class-action settlement, plaintiffs' attorneys
and the women they represent have every interest in getting
to court as quickly as possible.

AND WHAT ABOUT the scientific evidence? So far, several good epidemiologic studies have failed to show an association between

implants and a host of connective tissue diseases, symptoms, and abnormal lab tests.[10] The Women's Health Cohort Study found a relative risk of 1.2 that women with implants would *report* connective tissue disease, but the reports have not yet been validated. Although it is certainly possible that new studies might find a small association, enough is already known to say that a strong association is extremely unlikely. At most, breast implants could be a very weak risk factor for disease.

Let's assume, for purposes of discussion, that the relative risk turns out to be low—say, 1.2. What would that mean? The relative risk, as discussed earlier, simply indicates how high above the background level the risk is. In this case, it would be slightly elevated. For every 10 women *without* implants who develop connective tissue disease, 12 women *with* implants in an equal population would develop it. (For comparison, the relative risk of lung cancer among cigarette smokers is about 15; that is, for every 10 nonsmokers who develop lung cancer, 150 smokers do.) It is important to realize that we do not know exactly what a relative risk of 1.2 means for each of those 12 women who develop connective tissue disease. It could mean that in 2 of them, the implants were the sole cause of their disease and in the other 10 they played no role. Or it could mean that implants played a major role in 3 or 4 women and a very small one in the others. Or it could mean that implants contributed a varying amount to the disease in all 12. There is no way to know for sure on the basis of epidemiologic research. We would need to know more precisely *how* the implants contribute to or cause disease and why some women are more susceptible than others. Finding those answers would take a different sort of research—basic research and clinical studies. All we could say for sure with a relative risk of 1.2 is that, on *average,* implants contributed about 17 percent (0.2/1.2) to the disease. For any one woman among the 12, then, we could not say that but for the implants, she would not have developed the disease. Further, we would have to say that some other factor or group of factors was the dominant cause.

Now let's assume that the relative risk turns out to be 2.1 instead of 1.2 (although the present epidemiologic evidence indicates this level of risk would be extremely unlikely). What would that mean? For every 10 women *without* implants who develop connective tissue disease, 21 women *with* implants will develop it. Implants would therefore be more important than all other causes put together, since the relative risk would be more than double the background level. As in the example of a relative risk of 1.2, with a relative risk of 2.1 we would have no way of knowing the precise contribution of implants to connective tissue disease in each particular woman. They could be the sole cause in 11 and play no role in 10, or they could play a varying role in all of them. But we would know that, on *average,* they were the dominant cause, and so for any one woman, we could say that she would probably not have developed the disease if she had not received implants.

In fact, however, the epidemiologic studies to date have not found a relative risk of 2.1 and only one study—the largest, but likely to be biased because it was based on what women with implants said about their health after the FDA ban—has found a risk as high as 1.2. The best evidence now is a relative risk of 1.0, indicating no contribution of implants to disease. I assumed relative risks of 1.2 and 2.1 to illustrate a point— that is, that moving from a focus on the average results in a group of women to a focus on a *particular* woman is difficult. Nevertheless, unless we know something about individual susceptibilities, using the average as a proxy for the particular is the best we can do. And, from a scientific and logical perspective, it is the best the courts can do. Unfortunately, they have not done that, because of the way our judicial system works in tort cases.

As pointed out in Chapter 6, the courts are asked to make a judgment not about a population of women, but about an individual. For example, a court had to decide whether it was probable that implants caused Mariann Hopkins's mixed connective tissue disease.[11] At the time of the Hopkins case, there was no evidence of any increased risk, much less a relative risk greater than 2.0. Therefore, the only logical conclusion was that implants did not cause her disease. But the jury did not draw the logical conclusion. Instead, they attempted the impossible: to decide in the absence of evidence whether implants caused disease in a particular woman.

To a great extent, however, the courts have avoided the issue of causation altogether. Plaintiffs' attorneys have been remarkably successful in shifting the focus away from it. Instead of trying to demonstrate that the implants probably caused the plaintiff's disease, they simply assumed causation. They then focused on the manufacturers' behavior. Had they demonstrated safety? Were they negligent? Did they hide evidence? This shift in focus has received very little attention. Perhaps we are simply used to thinking of the controversy in terms of proven safety, because at the time of the FDA ban, attention was focused on whether safety had been demonstrated. Kessler was right in saying that from the FDA's viewpoint, the burden of proof was on the manufacturers. But in court, the burden of proof should be on the plaintiff. Can the plaintiff show that implants probably caused her disease? Since a torrent of lawsuits followed the FDA's decision, it may be that there was a natural tendency to assume that the basis for the decisions would be the same. Whatever the explanation, this

shift was pervasive, and it made the job of the plaintiffs' attorneys much easier.

Another shift taking place was in the nature of the harms
being attributed to breast implants. I have already discussed
the change in concerns from cancer to autoimmune or connective tissue disease, and then to "non-classic" disease.[12] As
the diseases became vaguer and harder to define, it became
increasingly difficult to study their association with implants.
Doctors who make their living diagnosing implant-related diseases and the lawyers who pay them have every reason to pos-
tulate increasingly obscure syndromes, as the well-defined
ones come under scientific scrutiny. To them, the best diseases
are those that can't be defined, because they can't be studied
systematically. A more reasonable shift was taking place at the
FDA. The agency was changing its major focus from systemic
diseases to local complications of implants. Kessler told Congress in August 1995, "We now have, for the first time, a reasonable assurance that silicone-gel implants do not cause a
large increase in traditional connective-tissue disease in
women."[13] He was now concerned primarily with the local
complications—contractures, leakage, rupture, and problems
with mammography. In justifying the continuation of the ban,
he rightly pointed out that just as we didn't know the risk of
systemic complications, we also didn't know the incidence of
local ones. Fortunately, this was an easier matter to study than
an ever-shifting constellation of nonspecific symptoms.

And who should do the research? When the FDA banned
breast implants, it was because the manufacturers had not fulfilled their obligation to produce evidence of safety. One way
for a company to do this is to fund research done by scientists
in established research institutions. In the case of breast implants, in particular, outside research is necessary, since

demonstrating safety requires large epidemiologic studies, which can only be conducted by epidemiologists who have access to large numbers of people. The manufacturers themselves do not have access to the subjects, nor do they have the expertise to carry out the studies. Since the ban, and under the prodding of the FDA, the manufacturers have begun to fund serious research into the safety of breast implants. This is the research they should have supported years before. Dow Corning, for example, contributed to the Mayo Clinic study through the American Society of Plastic and Reconstructive Surgeons' Educational Foundation. The company also supported the Women's Health Cohort Study. Funding such research was precisely what the FDA faulted the manufacturers for not doing earlier. Ironically, after the manufacturers began to fund research, plaintiffs' attorneys implied that the research was invalid for that very reason.[14] Surely, this was a Catch-22. The charge, however, did raise the larger issue of conflicts of interest in medical research. As government funding of research declines, more of it is supported by private industry. Does private support by a company with an interest in the drug or device under study automatically taint the research?

Much depends on how the research grant is given. Research institutions such as the Mayo Clinic and the Brigham and Women's Hospital (the Harvard hospital that houses the Nurses' Health Study and the Women's Health Cohort Study) have given a good deal of attention to preventing bias in privately funded research. They have established guidelines to prevent research from being influenced by a company that provides funding. First, the grant is customarily given to the institution, not to the researchers, so that the rules can be enforced. Full public disclosure of the source of funding is required. The company is usually not permitted to participate in the design of the study or in the analysis of the results. Often there is an agreement that the company will not be told about the results until the study is published or presented at a scientific meeting. Most important, there is usually an agreement that the results will be reported, regardless of the outcome. A recent study of the effects of large doses of vitamin A on pregnant women is a good example.[15] This study found vitamin A in high doses to cause birth defects. By prearranged agreement, the researchers reported these results, despite the fact that the study was funded by a manufacturer of vitamin supplements. Such precautions are necessary to prevent companies from distorting or withholding the results of research on their products. When the rules are followed, there is no reason to dismiss the study simply because it has been funded by a company with an interest in the outcome. (If there were, much of the biomedical research done in this country would have to be disregarded.)

Other countries have responded quite differently to the unfolding evidence about breast implants. Spain, for example, followed the lead of the FDA and banned breast implants in 1992, but lifted the ban later the same year, after reviewing the data.[16] The French Health Ministry can't seem to make up its mind. Like Spain, it followed the FDA's lead and pulled breast implants off the market in 1992. As the epidemiologic evidence accumulated, however, France reevaluated the situation, and in January 1995 lifted the ban.[17] Later the same year, they reinstituted it.[18] Great Britain chose to buck the trend altogether, and never followed the FDA's lead. The British Department of Health issued a report in 1993 saying they found no reason for a moratorium.[19] A 1994 update stated, "The conclusions from this updated analysis remain unchanged in that there remains no scientific evidence from the literature of any increased risk of connective tissue disease associated with silicone gel breast implants."[20] Committees established by the Canadian and French governments reached the same conclusion, as did the American Medical Association, the American Society of Plastic and Reconstructive Surgeons, and the American College of Rheumatology.

Whether the new evidence will lead the FDA to reverse its decision is unclear. The effect on the legal situation is also difficult to predict. Given Dow Corning's bankruptcy, the meltdown of the class-action settlement, and the precariousness of the new agreements with the other manufacturers, the legal situation may very well remain in flux for years. Adding to the complexity is the likelihood of a new rush to court now that Dow Chemical has been found liable for Dow Corning's implants in some jurisdictions. Although studies failing to find a link between implants and connective tissue disease, or studies finding only a weak link, may influence pending lawsuits, there is very little basis for optimism on that score. Almost certainly in this volatile situation, much will depend on public opinion.

WHATEVER THE END RESULT of the breast implant controversy, the story should give us all pause. Many people expect big business to be concerned primarily about profits and only as concerned about the safety of its customers as the law and public relations require. When I began looking into the breast implant story, I fully expected to find that the implant manufacturers fit this mold. What I was not prepared to find was the extent of the financial involvement of the plaintiffs' attorneys and the possible complicity of some physicians in their purposes. The derelictions of the manufacturers paled in comparison. As the breast implant story unfolded, three professions—law, medicine, and journalism—failed in their responsibilities to hold the controversy within the bounds of reason. The failure reflected certain underlying weaknesses within these professions. What were the problems revealed in each profession, and how might they be addressed?

The peculiar incentives within the legal profession are perhaps the most obvious problem. Our tort system enables lawyers to prey on people's fears, to destroy thriving companies, and, in the breast implant case, even to threaten an entire industry (medical devices) and an important area of medical research (epidemiologic studies)—and at the same time to make huge amounts of money in fees. The legal system virtually invites this sort of abuse. The practice of paying lawyers contingency fees in tort cases, along with the easy electronic exchange of information about lawsuits all over the country, means that plaintiffs' attorneys can mass-produce lawsuits of very little merit with almost no risk to themselves. If they win only one of every ten or twenty, they can still do very well. On the other hand, each lawsuit from every lawyer requires a response from the defendant. The costs of defending all the lawsuits can be very high, even if successful. Recall that DuPont spent $8 million successfully defending itself against lawsuits filed against it because it had supplied Teflon to the manufacturer of allegedly defective jaw implants. If a defendant loses just one of every ten or twenty cases, the costs can be enormous. Furthermore, losing just one lawsuit can stimulate an avalanche of others, and each loss usually means the stakes grow higher in the next case. Manufacturers therefore are usually eager to settle claims out of court, even when they believe the product has not caused the injury and they think they could *probably* win in court. Maybe contingency fees should be forbidden in this country, as they are elsewhere. At the very least, they should be much smaller than they are and perhaps restricted to clients who cannot afford a set fee.

The use of juries for tort cases is also problematic. Decisions by judges would almost certainly be sounder than those made by juries, because judges are educated to be dispassionate and to evaluate evidence. Many tort cases involve expert witnesses, who speak to fairly technical matters. To evaluate whether a product has caused a disease is difficult for nearly anyone. For a jury it is especially difficult, because its members usually have no competence in the area. They are often left to make judgments largely on the basis of the emotional appeals of the lawyers and their expert witnesses. Judges, too, may have no competence in the technical area, but they are much more resistant to lawyers' emotional appeals than juries usually are, and they can learn how to approach scientific questions—as, indeed, they are required to do by the Supreme Court in the *Daubert* decision (discussed in Chapter 6). The growing size of jury awards, especially punitive damages, also is problematic. Although judges often reduce the size of the damages after the verdict, large awards still create strong inflationary pressures. Other countries do not have jury trials for civil cases, and we should consider eliminating them for tort cases.

Other needed legal reforms should include some attention to the growing abuse of class actions as windfalls for attorneys. In addition, we should probably review the laws that permit suppliers of biomaterials to be sued for damages caused by products they had no part in designing or testing. Addressing these problems is important. But even more important, in my judgment, is to reform the way science is handled in the courtroom. If it were not for the nearly total lack of scientific standards in the breast implant cases, even a badly flawed legal system could not have worked such mischief. There is no reason that science in the courtroom cannot be as reliable as science elsewhere.

The most important reform we could make to raise scientific standards in the courtroom would be for judges to appoint expert witnesses, rather than to rely on witnesses hired by the opposing lawyers. Reputable experts could be recommended to courts by established scientific organizations, such as the National Academy of Sciences or the American Association for the Advancement of Science. These witnesses would be neutral—that is, they would represent neither side. In essence, they would interpret for the court the current scientific knowledge about the matter at hand. The task would be similar to the task of writing a review article for a journal. The experts would be expected to cite evidence from the scientific literature to support their interpretations. Although judges now have the option of appointing such witnesses, they rarely do so. The practice should be routine. And without reliable expert witnesses, science in the courtroom will continue to be a baffling mix of fact and speculation, of objectivity and self-interest. The verdicts will be no less baffling.

The breast implant story shows how courtroom procedure can ignore or misinterpret science. It also illustrates how the unrestrained use of subpoenas outside the courtroom can harass and even intimidate scientists engaged in research, to the detriment of all of us. The Mayo Clinic, for example, has collected medical information on the residents of Olmsted County for many decades. Because most patients in this relatively isolated, rural county receive their specialized medical care from the Mayo Clinic, the database (known as the Rochester Epidemiology Project) is not only huge, but comprehensive. And its yield has been prolific. Over 800 scientific studies on all sorts of medical questions have emanated from this one database. It is a unique resource. But it depends on the cooperation of the local doctors and their patients. When the plaintiffs' attorneys subpoenaed Sherine Gabriel for the records of all women in her study, as well as all who were considered for it, the Mayo Clinic was concerned that doctors, worried about maintaining the confidentiality of their patients, would withdraw from the Rochester Epidemiology Project. Similarly, the Nurses' Health Study is an ongoing study of some 100,000 women, which yields information about a wide range of medical questions, of which the effect of breast implants is only one. As in the case of the Rochester Epidemiology Project, subpoenas for the participants' records threaten confidentiality and therefore the existence of the database. Scientists working on both these projects are alarmed by this threat to their ability to continue their research. They are also worried about the time and effort involved in meeting what at least some of them perceive to be excessive and unreasonable demands for documents. If such concerns were to discourage further epidemiologic studies of breast implants, the plaintiffs' attorneys who have been largely responsible for issuing subpoenas for clinical records conceivably might have cause for satisfaction, but the rest of us should not.

Long-standing epidemiologic databases, such as those of the Rochester Epidemiology Project and the Nurses' Health Study, are all the more important because it would now be extremely difficult to assemble a new database to do research on breast implants. The reason is that the widespread publicity about breast implants since 1991 would color women's responses to questions about their health. Since women with breast implants have heard that the devices may cause all sorts of diseases and symptoms, it would be human nature for them to remember and magnify even ordinary complaints, as discussed earlier. Add to this unconscious tendency the fact that a great many women with implants have pending legal claims, and it becomes all but impossible to obtain unbiased information about their health. Even recent medical records could be biased. In contrast, studies based on the older databases considered only illnesses reported before a cutoff date (in the Mayo Clinic study, 1991; in the Nurses' Health Study, 1990).

What about the medical profession's role in this story? The lawyers could not exploit the breast implant controversy without the help of doctors who collect fees for making what are often dubious diagnoses. Not only are these doctors guilty of putting personal gain before their professional commitments, but they also subject women to unnecessary, costly, and sometimes risky treatments. Most doctors, to their credit, have resisted the temptation to join in the lucrative arrangement. Nevertheless, the medical profession as a whole bears some responsibility for the fact that a small group of doctors is able to get away with such blatantly unethical behavior. At least one of these doctors was reported to his state's Board of Medical Registration. When this book went to press, a year after the report, the board had still taken no action.

Finally, the media must share the blame for events in the early stages of the breast implant controversy. Despite the total lack of evidence, reporters were quite happy to feed and amplify the public's fascination with yet another health scare. There was little effort to provide a critical analysis of the issue, much less to put it in context. The public soon became utterly convinced that breast implants cause serious disease. It then exerted pressure on the FDA, which is necessarily a political body as well as a regulatory one. The FDA's advisory panels included advocates who were certain, despite the lack of evidence, that implants cause disease. Public hearings in this climate all but guaranteed the outcome. The legal system, whose

unscientific and outsized verdicts had largely initiated the
scare, then became the victim of the monster it created. With
each spectacular verdict, another was sure to follow, along
with a much larger number of out-of-court settlements. As the
Washington Post editorialized in the fall of 1995, "What's odd-
est about the implant situation at present is the continued di-
vergence between the results of medical studies (mandated by
the Food and Drug Administration when it took most implants off the market after its hearing in 1992) and the results
of legal proceedings unrelated to those hearings."[21] In trans-
mitting health news to the public, reporters have an obligation to be critical and to put any given story in its larger context. Too often they succumb to the temptation to fan fears.
And, unfortunately, that is all too easy to do. The breast implant controversy shows the proclivity of the public—unable
to tolerate uncertainty, unwilling to make minimal efforts to
evaluate scientific stories, and reinforced by the media—to
embrace uncritically the medical scare of the day.

Underlying the failings of the legal, medical, and jour-
nalistic professions in the breast implant story is the lure of financial gain. Lawyers become fabulously wealthy suing breast
implant manufacturers. Doctors and expert witnesses who cooperate with them share in some of the wealth. And the media
are often more interested in ratings and sales, which are parlayed into financial gain, than in responsible reporting. Many
members of these three professions pursue their private interests with utter disregard for the larger consequences. Even
the many healthy women with breast implants who now want
to take advantage of the furor over them are responding to the
lure of big financial awards. As Barry Schwartz points out in
his book, *The Costs of Living,* "Business is business, and the professions are business too."[22] But when all activities are based

on maximizing financial rewards, other considerations, including ethical standards, are lost. Money makes kings of rogues, sages of idiots, and heroes of thieves. A society too much in its thrall is left with no one to tend the public good.

The breast implant controversy shows every sign of continuing on its irrational course for years. Only an unyielding commitment to scientific evidence can stop it, and that does not seem very likely, given the money and passions involved. If all parties had accepted the discipline of evidence at the outset, the controversy would never have reached such proportions. It would hardly have gotten off the ground. But without a commitment to objective data, people were free to believe whatever they liked. Instead of basing their conclusions on the evidence, they willed the evidence to fit their favored conclusions. Do breast implants cause disease? If you were a plaintiffs' attorney, you would say they do. If you were a defense attorney, you would say they don't. Witnesses for both sides follow suit. Those who are critical of the supremacy of big business in American life would say they do. Those who believe that America's business *is* business would say they don't. This indifference to the need for evidence is a common thread in the many medical alarms that are sounded periodically in this country; the breast implant story simply illustrates it writ large. Whether or not breast implants are dangerous is not a question to be left to public opinion, corporate self-interest, and legal machinations. We ought to want to know the truth (or as near as we can come to it). But finding it requires careful scientific research and unbiased interpretation of the results. There are no shortcuts. Only by relying on scientific evidence can we hope to curb the greed, fear, and self-indulgence that too often govern such disputes. That is the lesson of the breast implant story.

NOTES

1: The Breast Implant Story

1. Estimates of the number of women with breast implants vary, but the FDA, in "Background Information on the Possible Health Risks of Silicone Breast Implants" (December 18, 1990; rev. February 8, 1991), says 2 million women in the United States "presently have" implants.

2. The 80 percent augmentation/20 percent reconstruction figure is used by almost everybody, including the FDA (in particular, the number appears in the June 1992 issue of the *FDA Consumer*). Also, Independent Advisory Committee on Silicone Gel-Filled Breast Implants, "Summary of the Report on Silicone-Gel-Filled Breast Implants," *Canadian Medical Association Journal*, 147 (1992):1141–46.

3. See D. Kessler, "The Basis for the FDA's Decision on Breast Implants," *New England Journal of Medicine*, 326 (1992):1713–15.

4. A few newspaper articles chronicles the stories of women who attempted to remove implants with razor blades. See W. Bunch, "Under the Knife: Woman Uses Razor to Remove Implants," *Newsday*, April 18, 1992, p. 7; also R. Bragg, "Desperation Forces Removal of Implants," *Houston Chronicle*, May 15, 1992, p. A1.

5. The explosion of breast implant cases in the courts was detailed in the following articles: B. Wiser, "Feud in Implant Settlement Stirs Debate over Tactics," *Washington Post*, May 11, 1994, p. D1; G. Kolata, "Details of Implant Settlement Announced by Federal Judge," *New York Times*, April 16, 1994, p. A16.

6. Juries bestowed several very large awards to breast implant recipients in the early 1990s. See W. Carlsen, "Jury Awards $7.3 Million in Implant Case," *San Francisco Chronicle,* December 14, 1991, p. A13; also "Record $25 Million Awarded in Silicone Implants Case," *New York Times,* December 24, 1992, p. A13.

7. Many of the local complications related to implants are detailed by Council on Scientific Affairs, American Medical Association, "Silicone Gel Breast Implants," *JAMA,* 270, no. 21 (December 1993): 2602–6. The FDA included risk information on these complications in the *Federal Register,* September 26, 1991:49098–99.

8. Information on breast implants and cancer risk can be found in Council on Scientific Affairs, American Medical Association, "Silicone Gel Breast Implants," *JAMA,* 270, no. 21 (December 1993):2602–6. See also D. M. Deapen and G. S. Brody, "Augmentation Mammaplasty and Breast Cancer: A 5-Year Update of the Los Angeles Study," *Plastic and Reconstructive Surgery,* 89, no. 4 (April 1992):660–65; D. M. Deapen et al., "The Relationship between Breast Cancer and Augmentation Mammaplasty: An Epidemiologic Study," *Plastic and Reconstructive Surgery,* 77, no. 3 (March 1986):361–68.

9. Details of the settlement were widely covered by the general media. See, for example, T. M. Burton, "U.S. Judge Clears Breast-Implant Accord," *Wall Street Journal,* September 2, 1994, p. B2. For full details, see the settlement notice, entitled "Proposed Breast Implant Litigation Settlement," which was distributed by the U.S. District Court of the Northern District of Alabama.

10. The first epidemiologic study of the possible link between breast implants and connective tissue disease was S. E. Gabriel et al., "Risk of Connective-Tissue Diseases and Other Disorders after Breast Implantation," *New England Journal of Medicine,* 330 (1994):1697–1702.

11. Norman Anderson is quoted in A. Frankel, "From Pioneers to Profits," *American Lawyer,* June 1992: 82.

2: Breast Implants

1. The increasing use of breast implants is detailed in S. E. Gabriel et al., "Trends in the Utilization of Silicone Breast Implants, 1964–1991, and Methodology for a Population-Based Study of Outcomes," *Journal of Clinical Epidemiology,* 48, no. 4 (April 1995):527–37.

2. Breast augmentation statistics, demographic material, and fee information come from the American Society of Plastic and Reconstructive Surgeons (Arlington Heights, Ill.), "1994 Plastic Surgery Statistics."

3. Changes in the pattern of breast implant use are discussed in J. Foreman, "Breast Implant Field Altered by FDA Edict," *Boston Globe,* March 13, 1994, p. A1; S. E. Gabriel et al., "Trends in the Utilization of Silicone Breast Implants, 1964–1991, and Methodology for a Population-Based Study of Outcomes," *Journal of Clinical Epidemiology,* 48, no. 4 (April 1995):527–37; Independent Advisory Committee on Silicone Gel-Filled Breast Implants, "Summary of the Report on Silicone-Gel-Filled Breast Implants," *Canadian Medical Association Journal,* 147 (1992):1141–46; and D. Hilzenrath, "Surviving the Breast-Implant Siege," *Washington Post,* June 24, 1994, p. F1.

4. Arthur Caplan quoted in J. Foreman, "Implants: Is Uninformed Consent a Woman's Right?" *Boston Globe,* January 13, 1992, p. 25.

5. See N. Wolf, *The Beauty Myth: How Images of Beauty Are Used against Women* (New York: William Morrow, 1991).

6. For more information about the history of breast augmentation and early silicone use see G. T. Grace and I. K. Cohen, "Silicones and Breast Surgery," in R. B. Noone (ed.), *Plastic and Reconstructive Surgery of the Breast* (Philadelphia: Mosby, 1991); E. H. Kopf, "Injectable Silicones," *Rocky Mountain Medical Journal,* 63 (1966):34–36; J. P.

Lalardie and R. Mouly, "History of Mammaplasty," *Aesthetic Plastic Surgery,* 2 (1978):167–76; and Council on Scientific Affairs, American Medical Association, "Silicone Gel Breast Implants," *JAMA,* 270, no. 21 (December 1993):2602–6.

7. For more information about the basic chemistry of silicone and its uses see S. A. Bradley, "The Use of Silicones in Plastic Surgery: A Retrospective View," *Plastic and Reconstructive Surgery,* 51 (1973):280–88; G. T. Grace and I. K. Cohen, "Silicones and Breast Surgery," in R. B. Noone (ed.), *Plastic and Reconstructive Surgery of the Breast* (Philadelphia: Mosby, 1991); and R. R. LeVier, M. C. Harrison, R. R. Cook, and T. H. Lane, "What Is Silicone?" *Plastic and Reconstructive Surgery,* 92 (1993):163–67.

8. Some of the side effects of injecting silicone directly into the breasts are documented in E. H. Kopf, C. A. Vinnik, J. J. Bongiovi, and D. J. Dombrowski, "Complications of Silicone Injections," *Rocky Mountain Medical Journal,* 73, no. 2 (1976):77–80.

9. Polyvinyl alcohol is discussed in G. T. Grace and I. K. Cohen, "Silicones and Breast Surgery," in R. B. Noone (ed.), *Plastic and Reconstructive Surgery of the Breast* (Philadelphia: Mosby, 1991).

10. More information about Cronin and Gerow's collaboration with Dow Corning on the first silicone-gel-filled breast implants can be found in S. A. Braley, "The Use of Silicones in Plastic Surgery: A Retrospective Review," *Plastic and Reconstructive Surgery,* 51, no. 3 (1973):280–88; J. P. Lalardie and R. Mouly, "History of Mammaplasty," *Aesthetic Plastic Surgery,* 2 (1978):167–76; and M. Swartz, "Silicone City," *Texas Monthly,* August 1995:65.

11. Suggested surgical procedures for augmentation mammaplasty were detailed by Dow Corning Corporation in a September 1976 bulletin (#51-266); also in T. D. Cronin and R. L. Greenberg, "Our Experiences with the Silastic Gel Breast Prosthesis," *Plastic and Reconstructive Surgery,* 46, no. 1 (1970):1.

12. Suggested surgical procedures for reconstruction after mastectomy are detailed in the U.S. Food and Drug Administration's publication "Breast Implants: An Information Update," June 1994 (rev. October 1994), Rockville, Md. See also R. H. Guthrie, *The Truth about Breast Implants* (New York: John Wiley & Sons, 1994).

13. Each of these problems is detailed in Council on Scientific Affairs, American Medical Association, "Silicone Gel Breast Implants," *JAMA,* 270, no. 21 (December 1993):2602–6. See also G. T. Grace and I. K. Cohen, "Silicones and Breast Surgery," in R. B. Noone (ed.), *Plastic and Reconstructive Surgery of the Breast* (Philadelphia: Mosby, 1991).

14. For years, implant manufacturers recommended that physicians perform this procedure. Closed capsulotomy was detailed in J. L. Baker, R. J. Bartels, and W. M. Douglas, "Closed Compression Technique for Rupturing a Contracted Capsule around a Breast Implant," *Plastic and Reconstructive Surgery,* 58, no. 2 (1976):137–41, and also in C. A. Vinnik, "Spherical Contracture of Fibrous Capsules around Breast Implants," *Plastic and Reconstructive Surgery,* 58, no. 5 (1976):555–60.

15. For more on complications from closed capsulotomy, see R. H. Guthrie, *The Truth about Breast Implants* (New York: John Wiley & Sons, 1994).

16. Estimates of rupture rates vary greatly. The general consensus among physicians, however, puts the rate at 4 to 6 percent. See Council on Scientific Affairs, American Medical Association, "Silicone Gel Breast Implants," *JAMA,* 270, no. (December (December 1993):2602–6; J. M. Destouet et al., "Screening Mammography in 350 Women with Breast Implants: Prevalence and Findings of Implant Complications," *American Journal of Radiology,* 159 (1992):973–78; and D. Kessler, "The Basis for the FDA's Decision on Breast Implants," *New England Journal of Medicine,* 326 (1992):1713–15.

17. Complications associated with polyurethane-coated implants are discussed in Independent Advisory Committee on Silicone Gel-Filled Breast Implants, "Summary of the Report on Silicone-Gel-Filled Breast Implants," *Canadian Medical Association Journal,* 147

(1992):1141–46; also C. S. Kasper, "Histologic Features of Breast Capsules Reflect Surface Configuration and Composition of Silicone Bag Implants," *American Journal of Clinical Pathology,* 102, no. 5 (1994):655–59.

18. Features of saline-filled and double-lumen implants are discussed in Independent Advisory Committee on Silicone Gel-Filled Breast Implants, "Summary of the Report on Silicone-Gel-Filled Breast Implants," *Canadian Medical Association Journal,* 147 (1992):1141–46.

19. Data about the prevalence of different types of implants are discussed in N. Handel et al., "Knowledge, Concern, and Satisfaction among Augmentation Mammaplasty Patients," *Annals of Plastic Surgery,* 30, no. 1 (1993):13–20, discussion 20–22.

20. A Swiss company, LipoMatrix, Inc., is conducting clinical trials on soybean-oil-filled implants. See "New Breast Implant to Be Tested in U.S.," *Boston Globe,* August 2, 1993, p. 48.

21. Complete transcripts of Jenny Jones's television programs from February 27 and March 30, 1992, are available from Burrelle's Information Services. Ms. Jones's story was featured in *People* magazine on March 2, 1992.

22. Mariel Hemingway's story is recounted in K. Muir, "Look Me in the Eyes and Tell Me They're Safe," *The Times* (London), May 7, 1994.

23. Information about the use of breast implants in Olmsted County can be found in S. E. Gabriel et al., "Trends in the Utilization of Silicone Breast Implants, 1964–1991, and Methodology for a Population-Based Study of Outcomes," *Journal of Clinical Epidemiology,* 48, no. 4 (April 1995):527–37.

24. Information about the 1990 survey is available from the American Society of Plastic and Reconstructive Surgeons (Arlington Heights, Ill.).

25. See N. Handel et al., "Knowledge, Concern, and Satisfaction among Augmentation Mammaplasty Patients," *Annals of Plastic Surgery,* 30, no. 1 (1993):13–20, discussion 20–22.

3: The FDA Ban on Implants

1. For a biographical sketch of Dr. David Kessler, see A. Gibbons, "Can David Kessler Revive the FDA?" and "New FDA Head: Profile of an Overachiever," both in *Science*, 252, no. 5003 (1991):200–3.

2. One comprehensive general chronology of the regulatory history of breast implants is R. Stombler, "Breast Implants and the FDA: Past, Present, and Future," *American College of Surgeons Bulletin,* June 1993:11–15. Dr. Kessler also recapped the history in his August 1, 1995, testimony before the Subcommittee on Human Resources and Intergovernmental Relations of the Committee on Government Reform and Oversight of the U.S. House of Representatives.

3. The very first of these reports, by K. Miyoshi et al., was published in a Japanese medical journal in 1964: "Hypergammaglobulinemia by Prolonged Adjuvanticity in Man: Disorders Developed after Augmentation Mammaplasty," *Japan Medical Journal*, 2122 (1964):9–14. Other reports from Japan of connective tissue diseases from injections of paraffin or silicone were published in American medical journals. See Y. Kumagai et al., "Scleroderma after Cosmetic Surgery: Four Cases of Human Adjuvant Disease," *Arthritis and Rheumatism*, 22, no. 5 (1979):532–37. Also Y. Kumagai et al., "Clinical Spectrum of Connective Tissue Disease after Cosmetic Surgery: Observations on 18 Patients and a Review of the Japanese Literature," *Arthritis and Rheumatism*, 27, no. 1 (1984):1–12.

4. See S. A. Van Nunen et al., "Post-Mammaplasty Connective Tissue Disease," *Arthritis and Rheumatism*, 25, no. 6 (1982):694–97.

5. The Stern verdict went out on the UPI wire on November 5, 1984, but was not widely reported in the general press. The case was revisited in 1992 by U. Thomas, "Woman's Breast Implant Suit Started the Dominoes," *Idaho Statesman*, March 14, 1992.

6. Dan Bolton's trip to Midland, Michigan, and the details about how and why the Dow Corning documents were sealed are recounted in A. Frankel, "From Pioneers to Profits," *American Lawyer,* June 1992:82.

7. Anderson first met Bolton at the November 1988 hearings, which Anderson chaired and where Bolton testified. See A. Frankel, "From Pioneers to Profits," *American Lawyer,* June 1992:82. See also P. Hilts, "Breast Implant Maker Accused on Data," *New York Times,* December 21, 1991, p. 8.

8. Sidney Wolfe's letter is cited in R. R. Cook et al., "The Breast Implant Controversy," *Arthritis and Rheumatism,* 37, no. 2 (1994):153–57.

9. A Frankel, "From Pioneers to Profits," *American Lawyer,* June 1992:82, notes Bolton's involvement with Public Citizen's breast implant clearinghouse.

10. For more on Command Trust Network, see C. Palmeri, "A Texas Gunslinger," *Forbes,* July 3, 1995:42–45.

11. See transcript of *Face to Face with Connie Chung,* December 10, 1990, available from Burrelle's Information Services.

12. Anderson and Goldrich are quoted in an Associated Press article describing the hearings. D. Mesce, "Breast Implant Controls Urged," AP, December 18, 1990.

13. For a full chronology of the regulatory process, see R. Strombler, "Breast Implants and the FDA: Past, Present, and Future," *American College of Surgeons Bulletin,* June 1993:11–15.

14. See N. Benac, "Companies Seek to Prove Breast Implants Are Safe," AP, June 10, 1991.

15. The FDA's reaction to the manufacturers' data was reported in P. J. Hilts, "Drug Agency Questions Companies' Safety Data on Breast Implants," *New York Times,* November 17, 1991, p. B6.

16. Proceedings of the November 12–14, 1991, FDA advisory panel are documented in Council on Scientific Affairs, American Medical Association, "Silicone Gel Breast Implants," *JAMA,* 270, no. 21 (December 1993):2602–6; "Breast Implant Use Allowed," *Facts on File World News Digest,* December 31, 1991, p. 993D1; R. Stombler, "Breast Implants and the FDA: Past, Present, and Future," *American College of Surgeons Bulletin,* June 1993:11–15; and Kessler's August 1, 1995, testimony to the Subcommittee on Human Resources and Intergovernmental Relations of the Committee on Government Reform and Oversight of the U.S. House of Representatives.

17. See W. Carlsen, "Jury Awards $7.3 Million in Implant Case," *San Francisco Chronicle,* December 14, 1991, p. A13.

18. See J. M. Adams, "Victim of Silicone Breast Implants Wants Value Placed on Women's Lives," *Chicago Tribune,* February 9, 1992, p. 21.

19. Several sources cited Bolton's reference to the secret documents during the Hopkins trial. See J. M. Adams, "Victim of Silicone Breast Implants Wants Value Placed on Women's Lives," *Chicago Tribune,* February 9, 1992, p. 21; M. McKee, "Breast Implant Maker Tries to Reopen Case," *The Recorder,* April 9, 1992, p. 1; and "Woman Wins Implant Suit," *New York Times,* December 17, 1991, p. A16.

20. Anderson and Bolton both tried to pressure the FDA to remove implants from the market. Their efforts are noted in A. Frankel, "From Pioneers to Profits," *American Lawyer,* June 1992:82; also in M. Gordon, "FDA Said to Have Reversed Policy after Seeing Secret Documents," AP, April 20, 1994.

21. Kessler recounted the events leading up to the January 6, 1992, moratorium in his August 1, 1995, testimony before the Subcommittee on Human Resources and Intergovernmental Relations of the Committee on Government Reform and Oversight of the U.S. House of Representatives. Also see Council on Scientific Affairs, American Medical Association, "Silicone Gel Breast Implants," *JAMA,* 270, no. 21 (December 1993):2602–6; P. J. Hilts, "Breast Implant Maker Accused on Data," *New York Times,* December 21, 1991, p. 8; and R. E. Stombler, "Breast Implants and the FDA: Past, Present, and Future," *American College of Surgeons Bulletin,* June 1993:11–15.

22. Kessler, in his August 1, 1995, congressional testimony, described the February 18–20, 1992, FDA advisory committee meeting. The status of Anderson at the meeting is discussed in R. L. Vernaci, "FDA Removes Doctor from Breast Implant Panel," AP, February 12, 1992; also in M. Cimons, "Member of FDA Breast Implant Advisory Committee Loses Vote," *Los Angeles Times,* February 13, 1992, p. A24. Anderson's later comments were made in a letter to Senator Herb Kohl in 1994. See M. Gordon, "FDA Said to Have Reversed Policy after Seeing Secret Documents," AP, April 20, 1994.

23. The panel's recommendations are detailed in R. E. Strombler, "Breast Implants and the FDA: Past, Present, and Future," *American College of Surgeons Bulletin,* June 1993:11–15. Kessler explained the decision, and the FDA's rationale, in "The Basis for the FDA's Decision on Breast Implants," *New England Journal of Medicine,* 326 (1992):1713–15.

24. See Dow Corning's package insert for the Silastic MSI mammary implant, p. 8 (1991).

25. The 800 pages of documents are available, for a fee, from Dow Corning.

26. See T. M. Burton, "Dow Corning Employees Falsified Data on Breast Implants, Counsel Concludes," *Wall Street Journal,* November 3, 1992, p. A3. Also B. Rensberger, "Breast Implant Records Were 'Faked.' " *Washington Post,* November 3, 1992, p. A3.

27. Dow Corning pulled out of the implant business in March 1992. See E. Neuffer, "Maker Quits Implant Market," *Boston Globe,* March March 1992, p. 1.

28. Mentor began its controlled study of implants in 1992. See "Silicone-Gel Breast Implants Resume with Restrictions," *Boston Globe,* November 4, 1992. Also U.S. Food and Drug Administration, "Breast Implants: An Information Update," June 1994 (rev. October 1994), Rockville, Md., p. 14.

29. The FDA announced the requirements for saline-filled implant PMAs in the *Federal Register,* January 8, 1993:3436–43. The regulatory process is explained in "Breast Implants: An Information Update," June 1994 (rev. October 1994), Rockville, Md., p. 16.

30. The FDA announced its proposed rule requiring premarketing approval for testicular prostheses in the *Federal Register*, January 13, 1993:4116–25. The final rule was published in the *Federal Register* on April 5, 1995 (pp. 1728–16).

31. See D. Kessler, "The Basis for the FDA's Decision on Breast Implants," *New England Journal of Medicine*, 326 (1992):1713–15.

32. See M. Angell, "Breast Implants: Protection or Paternalism?" *New England Journal of Medicine*, 326 (1992):1695–96.

33. For more on known risks from breast implants, see Chapter 2.

34. This quote, from Rosemary Locke, is taken from D. Mesce, "Breast Implant Controls Urged," AP, December 18, 1990.

35. See A. Fischer, "A Body to Die For," *Redbook*, September 1991:96.

36. See D. Kessler, "The Basis for the FDA's Decision on Breast Implants," *New England Journal of Medicine*, 326 (1992):1713–15.

37. For an example of this perspective, see J. Bovard, "Double-Crossing to Safety," *American Spectator*, January 1995: 24–29. See also M. Charen, "Save Us from the FDA," *Boston Globe*, December 29, 1994, p. 13.

38. Kessler's fight for regulatory authority over cigarettes peaked in the summer of 1995. See, for example, A. Devory and J. Schwartz, "FDA Given Power for Cigarette Rules," *Washington Post*, August 10, 1995, p. A1. Also G. Collins, "Companies Sue to Prevent Control of Cigarette Sales," *New York Times*, August 11, 1995, p. A18.

39. See Jenny Jones transcript, March 30, 1992, available from Burrelle's Information Services.

40. See N. Wolf, *The Beauty Myth: How Images of Beauty Are Used against Women* (New York: William Morrow, 1991), p. 245.

41. See J. Bovard, "Double-Crossing to Safety," *American Spectator*, January 1995: 24–29. See also M. Charen, "Save Us from the FDA," *Boston Globe*, December 29, 1994, p. 13.

4: The Rush to Court

1. See G. Kolata, "Details of Implant Settlement Announced," *New York Times,* April 5, 1994, p. A16. Also B. Wiser, "Feud in Implant Settlement Stirs Debate over Tactics," *Washington Post,* May 11, 1994, p. D1.

2. Barie S. Carmichael, Dow Corning corporate vice-president and executive director of corporate communications, cited this increase in an interview in the June 1995 issue of *TJFR Health News Reporter,* a monthly newsletter for health-care public relations specialists published in Ridgewood, N.J.

3. J. B. Weinstein, "Ethical Dilemmas in Mass Tort Litigation," 88 NW U.L. Rev 469, 480 (1994).

4. The display ad for Chandler, Franklin, and O'Brien appeared on p. 2 of the Health section of the July 26, 1994, *Washington Post.* Phone numbers for other plaintiffs' attorneys come from S. Torry, "Breast Implant Settlement Fund Sparks a Scramble," *Washington Post,* April 4, 1994, Business section, p. 7. See also T. Schroth, "Breast Implants: Latest Toxic Tort; Plaintiffs' Bar Launches Aggressive Drive for Clients," *New Jersey Law Journal,* April 13, 1992:1.

5. Details about the suits pending against Dow Corning come from the Q&A with Barie Carmichael (corporate vice-president and executive director of corporate communications) in the June 1995 issue of *TJFR Health News Reporter,* a monthly newsletter for health-care public relations specialists published in Ridgewood, N.J.

6. The membership increase to Public Citizen's breast implant clearinghouse is cited in A. Frankel, "From Pioneers to Profits," *American Lawyer,* June 1992: 82.

7. The growth of the ATLA breast implant group is cited in T. Schroth, "Breast Implants: Latest Toxic Tort; Plaintiffs' Bar

Launches Aggressive Drive for Clients," *New Jersey Law Journal,* April 13, 1992:1.

8. M. A. Glendon, *A Nation under Lawyers* (New York: Farrar, Straus & Giroux, 1994). For a scholarly treatment of tort law, see R. Epstein, *Cases and Materials on Torts,* 6th ed. (Boston: Little, Brown & Co., Law and Business Education, 1995).

9. For information about the number of civil suits filed annually in state and federal courts, see "Background" section of House of Representatives' Judiciary Committee Report (104–62) on HR-988, the Attorney Accountability Act of 1995.

10. For information about the number of tort cases, see *Facts and Trends* (a publication of the RAND Institute for Civil Justice), 3, no. 3 (spring 1995).

11. This modest growth, according to RAND (see note 10), is about 3 percent a year for state courts. In the federal courts, civil filings declined from 1985 to 1992, but began to increase once again in 1992.

12. See *Facts and Trends,* 3, no. 3 (spring 1995). Also E. C. Bassett, "The Litigation Explosion," *Journal of the Massachusetts Academy of Trial Attorneys,* 2, no. 4 (1995):16. Also D. J. Murphy, "When State Judges Are Elected," *Investor's Business Daily,* November 7, 1994, p. A1.

13. The increase in mass personal injury claims since 1980 is documented in D. Hensler and M. Peterson, "Understanding Mass Personal Injury Litigation: A Socio-Legal Analysis," *Brooklyn Law Review,* 59, no. 3 (1993):961–1063.

14. For more on trends in the use of punitive damage awards, see "Punitive Damages," *Facts and Trends,* 3, no. 3 (spring 1995).

15. Estimates of the increased total costs of the tort system between 1980 and 1990 come from D. J. Murphy, "When State Judges Are Elected," *Investor's Business Daily,* November 7, 1994, p. A1. The source cited by Murphy is Tillinghast, the insurance consulting unit of Towers Perrin.

16. The number of lawyers in the United States comes from the American Bar Association (personal communication). The 1980 (542,205) and 1991 (805,872) statistics are from *The Lawyer Statistical Report: The U.S. Legal Profession in the 1990s,* published by the American Bar Foundation. This source projected the lawyer population in 1995 to be 896,172. The ABA derived its own 1995 estimate of 896,140 from reports of licensing authorities in the 50 states.

17. See "Record $25 Million Awarded in Silicone Gel Implants Case," *New York Times,* December 24, 1992, p. A13.

18. The jury was informed of Dow Corning's value ($948 million) and instructed to keep it in mind when awarding punitive damages in the Hopkins case, according to Dow Corning's Petition for a Writ of Certiorari (note 4 on pp. 7–8).

19. See P. Brimelow and L. Spencer, "The Plaintiff Attorneys' Great Honey Rush," *Forbes,* October 16, 1989:197.

20. For more information about how the U.S. tort system differs from other countries' systems, see M. A. Glendon, *A Nation under Lawyers* (New York: Farrar, Straus & Giroux, 1994), p. 54.

21. See M. A. Glendon, *A Nation under Lawyers* (New York: Farrar, Straus & Giroux, 1994), p. 272.

22. Information about the history of asbestos in the courts is contained in D. Hensler and M. Peterson, "Understanding Mass Personal Litigation: A Socio-Legal Analysis," *Brooklyn Law Review,* 59, no. 3 (1993):961–1063 [1003–6]; the quote is on p. 961. See also D. Hensler, "A Glass Half Full, a Glass Half Empty: The Use of Alternative Dispute Resolution in Mass Personal Injury Litigation," *Texas Law Review,* 73 (1995):1587–1626.

23. For information about the history of DES in the courts, see D. Hensler and M. Peterson, "Understanding Mass Personal Litigation: A Socio-Legal Analysis," *Brooklyn Law Review,* 59, no. 3 (1993):961–1063 [981–82].

24. For information about the history of Bendectin in the courts, see D. Hensler and M. Peterson, "Understanding Mass Personal Litigation: A Socio-Legal Analysis," *Brooklyn Law Review*, 59, no. 3 (1993):961–1063 [978–81].

25. For information about the history of Dalkon Shield litigation, see D. Hensler and M. Peterson, "Understanding Mass Personal Litigation: A Socio-Legal Analysis," *Brooklyn Law Review*, 59, no. 3 (1993):961–1063 [983–86].

26. For more about the history of Agent Orange litigation, see D. Hensler and M. Peterson, "Understanding Mass Personal Litigation: A Socio-Legal Analysis," *Brooklyn Law Review*, 59, no. 3 (1993):961–1063 [1001–3].

27. For information about the litigation history of the Bjork-Shiley heart valve, see D. Hensler and M. Peterson, "Understanding Mass Personal Litigation: A Socio-Legal Analysis," *Brooklyn Law Review*, 59, no. 3 (1993):961–1063 [989–92].

28. See M. Purdy, "New York Girding for Surge in Suits over Lead Damage," *New York Times*, August 14, 1995, p. A1.

29. The effect of bankruptcy on litigation involving corporations like Johns-Manville and A. H. Robins received new attention after Dow Corning filed for bankruptcy. See S. Walsh, "Plaintiffs May Have Years to Wait in Implant Cases," *Washington Post*, May 16, 1995, p. A6; also S. Labaton, "Don't Sue, They Say. We Went Bankrupt," *New York Times*, May 21, 1995, p. E16. For more information about this, see D. Hensler and M. Peterson, "Understanding Mass Personal Injury Litigation: A Socio-Legal Analysis," *Brooklyn Law Review*, 59, no. 3 (1993):961–1063.

30. The increase in the use of class actions as a litigation tool starting in the 1970s is detailed in D. Hensler and M. Peterson, "Understanding Mass Personal Injury Litigation: A Socio-Legal Analysis," *Brooklyn Law Review*, 59, no. 3 (1993):961–1063. Also recapped in RAND Institute for Civil Justice Research Brief, January 1995.

31. Technical details of mass tort litigation—including class actions—are contained in *The Manual for Complex Litigation,* 3rd ed. (St. Paul, Minn.: Federal Judicial Center/West Publications, 1995).

32. See S. Torry, "Breast Implant Settlement Fund Sparks a Scramble," *Washington Post,* April 4, 1994, Business section, p. 7.

33. For more on lawsuits pending against the manufacturer of Norplant, see G. Kolata, "Will the Lawyers Kill Off Norplant?" *New York Times,* May 28, 1995, Sec. 3, p. 1.

34. See *The Manual for Complex Litigation,* 3rd ed. (St. Paul, Minn.: Federal Judicial Center/West Publications, 1995).

35. For more on the Judicial Panel on Multidistrict Litigation, see *The Manual for Complex Litigation,* 3rd ed. (St. Paul, Minn.: Federal Judicial Center/West Publications, 1995). Also *The Guide to American Law: Everyone's Legal Encyclopedia* (St. Paul, Minn.: West Publications, 1983), p. 389, and K. Jost, "Wrestling with Mass Torts," *The Recorder,* May 18, 1993, p. 1.

36. For more on Chesley and the genesis of the breast implant settlement, see H. Weinstein, "When Law, Tragedy Intersect," *Los Angeles Times,* March 26, 1994, p. A1. See also B. Wiser, "Feud in Implant Settlement Stirs Debate over Tactics," *Washington Post,* May 11, 1994, p. D1; A. Frankel, "Et tu, Stan?" *American Lawyer,* January/February 1994:68; and A. Blum, "Questions Raised on Class Action; Breast Implants," *National Law Journal,* March 30, 1992: 3.

37. See G. Kolata, "Details of Implant Settlement Announced by Federal Judge," *New York Times,* April 5, 1994, p. A16. Also *United States Law Week,* 62 USLW 2640 (April 19, 1994).

38. For complete details of the original settlement, see the "Settlement Notice," which Judge Sam Pointer's office sent with registration information to women with breast implants ("Proposed Breast Implant Litigation Settlement," U.S. District Court, Northern District of Alabama).

39. See D. Hilzenrath, "Renegotiation Order May Undo $4 Billion Implant Settlement," *Washington Post,* May 5, 1995, p. F1. Also D. R. Olmos and H. Weinstein, "Breast Implant Settlement in Peril," *Los Angeles Times,* May 5, 1995, p. A1.

40. Bolton's case against American Medical Systems was reported in S. Rosenfeld, "Penile Implant Maker Sued: Health Problems, Defects Concealed, Three Men Allege," *San Francisco Examiner,* May 21, 1994, p. A1.

41. Bolton is quoted in "California Class Action Filed over Penile Implants," *Liability Week,* 22, no. 9 (May 31, 1994).

42. Norplant's reliability, particularly for teenagers, was reported in M. Polaneczky et al., "Use of Levonergestrel Implants (Norplant) for Contraception in Adolescent Mothers," *New England Journal of Medicine,* 331 (1994):1201–6.

43. See G. Kolata, "Will the Lawyers Kill Off Norplant?" *New York Times,* May 28, 1995, Sec. 3, p. 1.

44. The feature of American law that allows people to make claims against any party involved in an allegedly harmful product is discussed by R. F. Service, "Liability Concerns Threaten Verdict in Implant Research," *Science,* 266, no. 5186 (1994):726–27.

45. The Vitek/DuPont case is discussed in "Implant Market a Minefield for Raw Material Suppliers," *Chemical Marketing Reporter,* 245, no. 22 May 30, (1994):20.

46. For more on the changing biomaterials market, see the Wilkerson Group's report, "Forces Reshaping the Performance and Contribution of the U.S. Medical Device Industry," prepared for the Health Industry Manufacturers' Association (Washington, D.C.), June 1995.

47. See L. Richwine, "Houston Dad Urges Legal Reforms," *Houston Chronicle,* May 21, 1994, Business section, p. 1.

48. Eleanor Gackstatter's testimony and Senator Lieberman's quote were reported in Bureau of National Affairs, Inc., "Senator to Seek

Changes in Product Liability Law" (Washington, D.C.: Daily Report for Executives, May 23, 1994, vol. 97: A2). See also L. Richwine, "Houston Dad Urges Legal Reforms," *Houston Chronicle*, May 21, 1994, Business section, p. 1.

49. This theory is discussed in B. J. Feder, "Implant Industry Is Facing Cutback by Top Suppliers," *New York Times*, April 25, 1994, p. A1.

50. For more background information on tort reform in Congress, see T. Gest, "Reversal of Fortunes," *U.S. News and World Report*, March 20, 1995:30; also "Is Lawsuit Reform Good for Consumers?" *Consumer Reports*, May 1995:312.

51. See G. McGovern, "Don't Reverse Medical Liability Reforms," *Christian Science Monitor*, August 22, 1994, p. 19.

52. See "America's Third Political Party: A Study of Political Contributions by the Plaintiff's Lawyer Industry," a report released by the American Tort Reform Association (Washington, D.C.), September 1994.

5: Scientific Evidence

1. For more information about the design and analysis of studies, see C. H. Hennekens, J. E. Buring, and S. L. Mayrent (eds.), *Epidemiology in Medicine* (Boston: Little, Brown, 1987), pp. 244–46.

2. The peer-review process for the *New England Journal of Medicine* is described in detail in "The Journal's Peer Review Process," *New England Journal of Medicine*, 321 (1989):837–39.

3. The cold fusion incident became the subject of a book by science journalist Gary Taubes. See G. Taubes, *Bad Science: The Short Life and Hard Times of Cold Fusion* (New York: Random House, 1993).

4. For a general discussion of risks, see R. L. Keeney, "Decisions about Life-Threatening Risks," *New England Journal of Medicine,* 331 (1994):193–96.

5. This material is presented in more detail in M. Angell, "The Interpretation of Epidemiologic Studies," *New England Journal of Medicine,* 323 (1990):823–25. For a broader discussion of epidemiologic research, see G. Taubes, "Epidemiology Faces Its Limits," *Science,* 269 (July 14, 1995):164–69.

6. See S. E. Gabriel et al., "Risk of Connective-Tissue Diseases and Other Disorders after Breast Implantation," *New England Journal of Medicine,* 330 (1994):1697–1702.

7. See C. H. Hennekens et al., "Self-Reported Breast Implants and Connective Tissue Diseases in ⌐ nale Health Professionals," *Journal of the American Medical Association,* 275 (1996): 616–21.

8. This study is known as the Nurses' Health Study. See J. Sanchez-Guerrero et al., "Silicone Breast Implants and the Risk of Connective-Tissue Diseases and Symptoms," *New England Journal of Medicine,* 332 (1995):1666–70.

9. See H. J. Englert and P. Brooks, "Scleroderma and Augmentation Mammoplasty—A Causal Relationship?" *Australia and New Zealand Medical Journal,* 24 (1994):74–80, and M. C. Hochberg et al., "Frequency of Augmentation Mammoplasty in Patients with Systemic Sclerosis: Data from the Johns Hopkins–University of Maryland Scleroderma Center," *Journal of Clinical Epidemiology,* 48, no. 4 (April 1995):565–69.

10. For a list of controlled epidemiologic studies of the question, see S. E. Gabriel et al., "Trends in the Utilization of Silicone Breast Implants, 1964–1991, and Methodology for a Population-Based Study of Outcomes," *Journal of Clinical Epidemiology,* 48 (1995):535.

11. This study was published in a Japanese medical journal. See K. Miyoshi et al., "Hypergammaglobulinemia by Prolonged Adjuvanticity in Man: Disorders Developed after Augmentation Mammaplasty," *Japan Medical Journal,* 2122 (1964):9–14.

12. These studies of directly injected silicone, published in U.S. medical journals, are Y. Kumagai et al., "Scleroderma after Cosmetic Surgery: Four Cases of Human Adjuvant Disease," *Arthritis and Rheumatism,* 22, no. 5 (1979):532–37; Y. Kumagai et al., "Clinical Spectrum of Connective Tissue Disease after Cosmetic Surgery: Observations on 18 Patients and a Review of the Japanese Literature," *Arthritis and Rheumatism,* 27, no. 1 (1984):1–12.

13. This first paper, linking silicone-gel-filled breast implants and connective tissue disease, was S. A. Van Nunen et al., "Post-Mammaplasty Connective Tissue Disease," *Arthritis and Rheumatism,* 25, no. 6 (1982):694–97.

14. F. B. Vasey, M. D., and J. Feldstein, *The Silicone Breast Implant Controversy* (Freedom, Calif.: The Crossing Press, 1993), p. 55.

15. The dog studies described here were the subject of widespread speculation when Dow Corning released 800 pages of internal documents in 1992. For example, see the transcript of ABC's *Primetime Live* for February 13, 1992, available from Nexis. See also A. Frankel, "From Pioneers to Profits," *American Lawyer,* June 1992:82.

16. See N. Kossovsky, "Immunology of Silicone Breast Implants," *Journal of Biomaterials Applications,* 8 (1994):237–46. Also N. Kossovsky, "Surface Dependent Antigens Identified by High Binding Avidity of Serum Antibodies in a Subpopulation of Patients with Breast Implants," *Journal of Applied Biomaterials,* 4 (1993):281–88.

17. See M. Lappé, "Silicone-Reactive Disorder: A New Autoimmune Disease Caused by Immunostimulation and Superantigens," *Medical Hypotheses,* 41 (1993):348–52.

18. See D. M. Gott and J. J. B. Tinkler, "Evaluation of Evidence for an Association between the Implantation of Silicones and

Connective Tissue Disease: Data Published from the End of 1991 to July 1994" (London: Medical Devices Directorate, December 1994).

6: Science in the Courtroom

1. See A. Frankel, "From Pioneers to Profits," *American Lawyer,* June 1992:82.

2. For a fuller analysis, see B. Black, "Matching Evidence about Clustered Health Events with Tort Law Requirements," *American Journal of Epidemiology,* 132 (1990):579–86.

3. For more information on the role of expert testimony in the courtroom, see L. Loevinger, "Science as Evidence," *Jurimetrics Journal,* winter 1995:153–90. Also B. Black, "Evolving Legal Standards for the Admissibility of Scientific Evidence," *Science,* 239, no. 4847 (1988):1508–12.

4. See A. Frankel, "From Pioneers to Profits," *American Lawyer,* June 1992:82.

5. Biographical details about Mariann Hopkins, and the case chronology, primarily come from two sources: the decision of the United States Court of Appeals for the 9th Circuit, August 26, 1994 (*Mariann Hopkins v. Dow Corning Corp.* 33F.3d 1116 1994), and the Petition for a Writ of Certiorari to the U.S. Supreme Court (*Dow Corning v. Mariann Hopkins,* No. 94-861, 1994). See also J. M. Adams, "Victim of Silicone Breast Implants Wants Value Placed on Women's Lives," *Chicago Tribune,* February 9, 1992, p. 21.

6. Hopkin quotes are taken from J. M. Adams, "Victim of Silicone Breast Implants Wants Value Placed on Women's Lives," *Chicago Tribune,* February 9, 1992, p. 21, and A. Frankel, "From Pioneers to Profits," *American Lawyer,* June 1992:82.

7. See A. Frankel, "From Pioneers to Profits," *American Lawyer,* June 1992:82.

8. See D. M. Gott and J. J. B. Tinkler, "Evaluation of Evidence for an Association between the Implantation of Silicones and Connective Tissue Disease: Data Published from the End of 1991 to July 1994" (London: Medical Devices Directorate, December 1994).

9. See M. Lappé, *Chemical Deception: The Toxic Threat to Health and the Environment* (San Francisco: Sierra Club, 1991).

10. Kossovsky's credentials are documented in the *Official ABMS Directory of Board Certified Medical Specialists,* 27th ed. (Philadelphia: Reed Reference Publishing, 1995).

11. Vasey's credentials are documented in the *Official ABMS Directory of Board Certified Medical Specialists,* 27th ed. (Philadelphia: Reed Reference Publishing, 1995).

12. For Vasey's position, see his book, F. B. Vasey and J. Feldstein, *The Silicone Breast Implant Controversy: What Women Need to Know* (Freedom, Calif.: Crossing Press, 1993).

13. The verdict was widely publicized. See, for example, W. Carlsen, "Jury Awards $7.3 Million in Implant Case," *San Francisco Chronicle,* December 14, 1991, p. A13, and J. M. Adams, "Victim of Silicone Breast Implants Wants Value Placed on Women's Lives," *Chicago Tribune,* February 9, 1992, p. 21. See also the decision of the United States Court of Appeals for the 9th Circuit, August 26, 1994 (*Mariann Hopkins v. Dow Corning Corp.* 33F.3d 1116 1994).

14. Dow Corning announced it was pulling out of the breast implant market in March 1992. See E. Neuffer, "Maker Quits Implant Market," *Boston Globe,* March 20, 1992, p. 1.

15. See the decision of the United States Court of Appeals for the 9th Circuit, August 26, 1994 (*Mariann Hopkins v. Dow Corning Corp.* 33F.3d 1116 1994).

10. For information about how the Johnson verdict affected O'Quinn's breast implant case load, see "Record $25 Million Awarded in Silicone Gel Implants Case," *New York Times*, December 24, 1992, p. A13. See also G. Taylor, "Breast Implant Suits Pouring In after $25 Million Verdict," *National Law Journal*, January 18, 1993:3.

11. See P. Brimelow and L. Spencer, "The Best Paid Lawyers in America" and "The Top Ten," *Forbes*, October 16, 1989:197, 204.

12. O'Quinn's 2,000-plus breast implant clients are often cited in the media. See G. Kolata, "Legal System and Science Come to Differing Conclusions on Silicone," *New York Times*, May 16, 1995, p. D6. See also M. McKee, "Deadline Looms for Implant Makers," *The Recorder*, September 9, 1994, p. 1, and C. Palmeri, "A Texas Gunslinger," *Forbes*, July 3, 1995:42–45.

13. See O'Quinn's comments in C. Palmeri, "A Texas Gunslinger," *Forbes*, July 3, 1995:42–45.

14. Information from Richard Laminack about the number of cases settled out of court (500) and the percentage referred by other lawyers (70 percent) comes from C. Palmeri, "A Texas Gunslinger," *Forbes*, July 3, 1995:42–45.

15. O'Quinn's average out-of-court settlement is noted in J. Nocera, "Fatal Litigation" (Part 2), *Fortune*, October 23, 1995:138.

16. O'Quinn's personal worth is cited in J. Nocera, "Fatal Litigation" (Part 1), *Fortune*, October 16, 1995:60–82.

17. "State the Case Simply by Starting with Voir Dire," *National Law Journal*, February 8, 1993:S-10.

18. These accusations were outlined in M. McKee, "Timing Is Everything," *The Recorder*, July 8, 1994, p. 1.

19. Dr. Sherine Gabriel first presented her findings at the annual meeting of the American College of Rheumatology, San Antonio, Texas, November 7–11, 1993.

20. See G. Kolata, "Legal System and Science Come to Differing Conclusions on Silicone," *New York Times,* May 16, 1995, p. D6.

21. See "About 14,700 Women Leave Implant Deal," *Wall Street Journal,* July 25, 1994, p. B4. See also B. Sapino, "Houston Threatens $4.25B Implant Deal," *Texas Lawyer,* August 1, 1994, p. 1.

22. The lack of campaign contribution limits in Texas is discussed (in the context of new limits on the length of campaigns) in J. D. Montgomery, "Reforming Judicial Elections: State Supreme Court Has Ordered a Step in the Right Direction," *Houston Post,* November 13, 1994, p. C1.

23. Tactics to solicit breast implant clients were detailed in R. Connelly, "From Flood to Deluge in Breast-Implant Cases: Houston's Hot in Latest Mass Tort Craze," *Texas Lawyer,* January 11, 1993:1.

24. Texas plaintiffs' attorneys are specifically mentioned in G. Kolata, "Will the Lawyers Kill Off Norplant?" *New York Times,* May 28, 1995, Sec. 3, p. 1. See also "Breast Implants and Norplant: The Silicone Connection," *Medical-Legal Aspects of Breast Implants,* 3, no. 7 (1995):1.

25. Two investigative reports by TV journalists have examined how doctors work with lawyers on implant cases. The first, by John Getter of KHOU in Houston, was broadcast on October 10, 1994. The second, broadcast on CNN on October 16, 1994, called "The Merchants of Fear," was part of a CNN series called *Fire and Fury.*

26. O'Quinn's run-in with the Texas bar association was widely reported. See P. Brimelow and L. Spencer, "The Best Paid Lawyers in America" and "The Top Ten," *Forbes,* October 16, 1989:197, 204. See also P. Burka, "Taking the Law into His Own Hands: John O'Quinn," *Texas Monthly,* September 1994:109. Information about O'Quinn's public reprimand can be confirmed by the Texas State Bar in Austin, telephone number (512)463-1463.

27. For more on physicians' roles, see G. Kolata and B. Meier, "Implant Lawsuits Create a Medical Rush to Cash In," *New York Times,* September 18, 1995, p. A1.

28. Lewy's point of view is represented in his public education brochure, "Frequently Asked Questions from Breast Implant Research" (Houston: Breast Implant Research, Inc., 1994).

29. For more on Lewy's practice and income, see G. Kolata and B. Meier, "Implant Lawsuits Create a Medical Rush to Cash In," *New York Times,* September 18, 1995, p. A1.

30. This report by John Getter of KHOU in Houston was broadcast on October 10, 1994.

31. This CNN report, *Fire and Fury,* Part 4: "The Merchants of Fear," was broadcast on October 16, 1994.

32. See "Breast Implant Witnesses Can Find Themselves Facing Conflicts of Interest," *Medical-Legal Aspects of Breast Implants,* 3, no. 5 (April 1995):8.

33. For details about Nir Kossovsky's company, SBI Laboratories, see G. Taubes, "Silicone in the System," *Discover,* December 1995:65–75.

34. Kossovsky's disagreement with the FDA is detailed in the CNN report *Fire and Fury,* Part 4: "The Merchants of Fear," broadcast on October 16, 1994.

8: Americans and Health News

1. Sidney Wolfe's involvement in the breast implant story is discussed in Chapter 3.

2. For a discussion of American paranoia, see M. Kelly, "The Road to Paranoia," *New Yorker,* June 19, 1995:60–75.

3. For examples of this genre of self-help health books, see D. Chopra, *Quantum Healing: Exploring the Frontiers of Mind, Body, Medicine* (New York: Bantam, 1990); D. Chopra, *Ageless Body, Timeless Mind* (New York: Crown, 1993); B. S. Seigel, *Peace, Love and Healing: The Bodymind and the Path to Self-Healing—An Exploration* (New

York: HarperCollins, 1989); B. Siegel, *Love, Medicine, and Miracles* (New York: HarperCollins, 1986); and A. Weil, *Spontaneous Healing: How to Enlist and Enhance the Body's Own Gifts for Maintaining and Healing Itself* (New York: Knopf, 1995).

4. For more on the anti-science sentiment, see Chapter 9.

5. See E. L. Bierman, "Atherosclerosis and Other Forms of Arteriosclerosis," in K. J. Isselbacher et al. (eds.), *Harrison's Principles of Internal Medicine,* 13th ed. (New York: McGraw-Hill, 1994), p. 1106; R. Benfante et al., "Elevated Serum Cholesterol Is a Risk Factor for Both Coronary Heart Disease and Thromboembolic Stroke in Hawaiian Japanese Men: Implications of Shared Risk," *Stroke,* 25 (1994):814–20; and J. Pekkanen et al., "Ten-Year Mortality from Cardiovascular Disease in Relation to Cholesterol Level among Men with and without Preexisting Cardiovascular Disease," *New England Journal of Medicine,* 322 (1990):1700–7.

6. See W. C. Willett and A. Ascherio, "Trans Fatty Acids: Are the Effects Only Marginal?" *American Journal of Public Health,* 84 (1994):722–24.

7. Studies on the beneficial effects of oat bran include R. W. Kirby et al., "Oat-Bran Intake Selectively Lowers Serum Low-Density Lipoprotein Cholesterol Concentrations on Hypercholesterolemic Men," *American Journal of Clinical Nutrition,* 43 (1981):824–29, and J. W. Anderson et al., "Hypocholesterolemic Effects of Oat-Bran or Bean Intake for Hypercholesterolemic Men," *American Journal of Clinical Nutrition,* 40 (1984):1146–55.

8. A study showing no beneficial effects for oat bran is J. F. Swain et al., "Comparison of the Effects of Oat Bran and Low-Fiber Wheat on Serum Lipoprotein Levels and Blood Pressure," *New England Journal of Medicine,* 322 (1990):147–52.

9. A study showing a correlation between saccharin and bladder cancer is G. R. Howe et al., "Artificial Sweeteners and Human Bladder Cancer," *Lancet,* 2 (1977):578–81.

10. A study showing saccharin doesn't cause bladder cancer is R. N. Hoover and P. H. Strasser, "Artificial Sweeteners and Human Bladder Cancer: Preliminary Results," *Lancet,* 1 (1980):837–40.

11. Studies showing beneficial effects of antioxidants are M. J. Stampfer et al., "Vitamin E Consumption and the Risk of Coronary Disease in Women," *New England Journal of Medicine,* 328 (1993):1444–49; E. B. Rimm et al., "Vitamin E Consumption and the Risk of Coronary Heart Disease in Men," *New England Journal of Medicine,* 328 (1993):1450–56; R. M. Bostick et al., "Reduced Risk of Colon Cancer with High Intake of Vitamin E: The Iowa Women's Health Study," *Cancer Research,* 52 (1993):4230–37; and L. Roncucci et al., "Antioxidant Vitamins or Lactulose for the Prevention of the Recurrence of Colorectal Adenomas," *Diseases of the Colon and Rectum,* 36 (1993):227–34.

12. A study showing antioxidants could be bad for you is Alpha-Tocopherol, Beta Carotene Cancer Prevention Study Group, "The Effect of Vitamin E and Beta Carotene on the Incidence of Lung Cancer and Other Cancers in Male Smokers," *New England Journal of Medicine,* 330 (1994):1029–35.

13. See B. Armstrong et al., "Association between Exposure to Pulsed Electromagnetic Fields and Cancer in Electric Utility Workers in Quebec, Canada, and France," *American Journal of Epidemiology,* 140 (1994):805–20.

14. See D. A. Savitz and D. P. Loomis, "Magnetic Field Exposure in Relation to Leukemia and Brain Cancer Mortality among Electrical Utility Workers," *American Journal of Epidemiology,* 141 (1995):123–34.

15. The study showing that postmenopausal estrogen increases the risk of breast cancer is G. A. Colditz et al., "The Use of Estrogens and Progestins and the Risk of Breast Cancer in Postmenopausal Women," *New England Journal of Medicine,* 332 (1995):1589–93.

16. The study showing no increase of breast cancer with postmenopausal estrogen is J. L. Stanford et al., "Combined Estrogen and

Progestin Hormone Replacement Therapy in Relation to Risk of Breast Cancer in Middle-Aged Women," *JAMA,* 274 (1995):137–42.

17. See "Diet Roulette," *New York Times,* May 20, 1994, p. A26.

18. Ellen Goodman's column appeared in the *Boston Globe* on April 17, 1994, p. A27.

19. See E. Giovannucci et al., "A Retrospective Cohort Study of Vasectomy and Prostate Cancer in U.S. Men," *JAMA,* 269 (1993):878–82.

20. G. A. Colditz et al., "The Use of Estrogens and Progestins and the Risk of Breast Cancer in Post-Menopausal Women," *New England Journal of Medicine,* 332 (1995):1589–93.

21. For further reading on epidemiology, see C. H. Hennekens, J. E. Buring, and S. L. Mayrent (eds.), *Epidemiology in Medicine* (Boston: Little, Brown, 1987), pp. 244–46.

22. The cold fusion incident is detailed by Gary Taubes in *Bad Science: The Short Life and Hard Times of Cold Fusion* (New York: Random House, 1993).

23. The coffee-and-pancreatic-cancer study cited is B. MacMahon et al., "Coffee and Cancer of the Pancreas," *New England Journal of Medicine,* 304 (1981):630–33.

24. For examples of the media treatment given to the coffee-and-pancreatic-cancer study, see H. M. Schmeck, "Study Links Coffee Use to Pancreas Cancer," *New York Times,* March 12, 1981, p. B15; "Coffee Nerves: Is There Cancer in the Cup?" *Time,* March 23, 1981:73; M. Clark and P. Malmaud, "Coffee—A Cancer Culprit?" *Newsweek,* March 23, 1981:87; and M. Sinclair, "America's Favorite Pick-Me-Up Comes under Fire," *Washington Post,* March 23, 1981, p. A1.

25. The original group of authors revisited and revised their findings in 1986. See C.-C. Hsieh et al., "Coffee and Pancreatic Cancer (Chapter 2)," *New England Journal of Medicine,* 315 (1986):587–89. This correction was not as widely reported as the 1981 study. Typical treatment included that of the *Chicago Tribune,* which ran a wire-service story ("Coffee Link to Cancer Questioned," August 29, 1986, p. 4), and the *Los Angeles Times* ("Drink Up: New Research Disputes Reported Link between Coffee, Cancer," August 31, 1986, Metro, Part 2, p. 4).

26. See GUSTO Investigators, "An International Randomized Trial Comparing Four Thrombolytic Strategies for Acute Myocardial Infarction," *New England Journal of Medicine,* 329 (199):673–82.

27. B. A. Lehman, "Cancer Drug Is Found to Have Heart Benefit: Anti-Clotting Therapy Found to Spare Lives," *Boston Globe,* September 2, 1993, p. 3.

28. Lipid Research Clinics Program, "The Lipid Research Clinics Coronary Primary Prevention Trial Results. I. Reduction in the Incidence of Coronary Heart Disease," *JAMA,* 251 (1984):351–64.

29. Rates for 10-year risk of death from cardiovascular disease come from J. Pekkanen et al., "Ten-Year Mortality from Cardiovascular Disease in Relation to Cholesterol Level among Men with and without Preexisting Cardiovascular Disease," *New England Journal of Medicine,* 322 (1990):1700–7.

30. For general arguments about risk see R. L. Keeney, "Decisions about Life-Threatening Risks," *New England Journal of Medicine,* 331 (1994):193–96. Also P. E. Ross, "Lies, Damned Lies and Medical Statistics," *Forbes,* August 14, 1995:130–35.

9: Breast Implants and the Rejection of Science

1. See C. Sagan, "Wonder and Skepticism," *Skeptical Inquirer,* 19, no. 1 (January/February 1995):24–30.

2. See P. Gross and N. Levitt, *Higher Superstition: The Academic Left and Its Quarrels with Science* (Baltimore: Johns Hopkins University Press, 1994).

3. For more on Afrocentric science, see J. Travis, "Clashing Cultures: Schools Stumble on an Afrocentric Science Essay," *Science,* 262 (November 12, 1993):1121–22.

4. For an example of a backlash against science by environmentalists, see K. Sale, "Setting Limits on Technology," *The Nation,* 260, no. 22 (June 5, 1995):785.

5. The most infamous example of such an individual is the Unabomber, whose bombing campaign—begun in 1978—has resulted in 3 deaths and 16 injuries. This individual's 35,000-word manifesto, "Industrial Society and Its Future," was published in the *Washington Post* on September 19, 1995.

6. Sidney Wolfe's involvement in the breast implant controversy is discussed in Chapter 3.

7. See S. Harding, *The Science Question in Feminism* (Ithaca: Cornell University Press, 1986).

8. See M. F. Belenky et al., *Women's Ways of Knowing: Development of Self, Voice, and Mind* (New York: Basic Books, 1986).

9. See B. Rensberger, "Flabulous Discovery! Drug Found that Burns Fat in Mice; Human Test Next," *Washington Post,* July 27, 1995, p. A1.

10. This attitude is exemplified by Margaret Branch, an Albuquerque lawyer, who says her breast implant practice allows her "to do something about our health care for women in this country"; quoted in K. S. Hirsh, "Storm Warning: Breast-Implant Lawsuits Approach Flood Stage," *Chicago Tribune,* January 10, 1993, Womanews, p. 9. Other lawyers interviewed in the article concur.

11. See J. E. Mack, *Abduction: Human Encounters with Aliens* (New York: Macmillan [Charles Scribner's Sons], 1994).

12. Mack is quoted in T. Genoni, "Exploring Mind, Memory, and the Psychology of Belief," *Skeptical Inquirer,* 19, no. 1 (January/February 1995):10–13.

13. Wittgenstein quote is from his *Philosophical Investigations,* 3d ed. (New York: Macmillan, 1968), Part 1, Section 109.

14. For a discussion of daytime talk shows and the paranormal, see C. E. Emery, "Tales from the TV Talk Shows," *Skeptical Inquirer*, 19, no. 3 (May/June 1995):12–13.

15. See D. Eisenberg, " 'Nonconventional' Medicine in the United States—Prevalence, Costs and Patterns of Use: Results of a National Survey," *New England Journal of Medicine*, 328 (1993):246–52.

16. For a summary of the controversy surrounding the NIH's Office of Alternative Medicine, see E. Marshall, "The Politics of Alternative Medicine," *Science*, 265 (September 30, 1994):2000–2.

17. For more on the current state of homeopathy, see J. Foreman, "Homeopathy Makes No Sense but Science Takes a Look Anyway," *Boston Globe*, July 17, 1995, p. 25.

18. See R. L. Park, "The Danger of Voodoo Science," *New York Times*, July 9, 1995, Sec. 4, p. 15, and C. H. Sommers, "The Flight from Science and Reason," *Wall Street Journal*, July 10, 1995, p. A14.

19. See R. L. Park, "The Danger of Voodoo Science," *New York Times*, July 9, 1995, Sec. 4, p. 15.

20. See C. Sagan, "Wonder and Skepticism," *Skeptical Inquirer*, 19, no. 1 (January/February 1995):24–30.

21. Risks from Bendectin, asbestos, and radon are discussed in K. R. Foster, D. E. Bernstein, and P. W. Huber (eds.), *Phantom Risk: Scientific Inference and the Law* (Cambridge: MIT Press, 1993). Gulf War syndrome is discussed in A. Pine, "Government Study of Veterans Finds No Evidence of a 'Gulf War' Disease," *Los Angeles Times*, August 2, 1995, p. A10.

10: Where We Stand . . .
and for How Long

1. See T. Burton, "Implant Fund Is Too Small to Cover Claims," *Wall Street Journal*, May 2, 1995, p. A3. Also D. R. Olmos and H. Weinstein,

"Breast Implant Settlement in Peril," *Los Angeles Times,* May 5, 1995, p. A1.

2. See "Proposed Breast Implant Litigation Settlement," which was prepared and distributed by the U.S. District Court, Northern District of Alabama.

3. As of June 1, 1995, 248,500 women had submitted claims for current illness under the terms of the settlement, according to the July 31, 1995, message on Judge Pointer's recorded settlement information line (800-887-6828).

4. See "Money Shortage Looms in Implant Case," *New York Times,* June 17, 1995, p. 8.

5. See D. S. Hilzenrath, "Renegotiation Order May Undo $4 Billion Implant Settlement," *Washington Post,* May 5, 1995, p. F1.

6. See B. Meier, "Implant Pact in Jeopardy as Lawyers Miss Deadline," *New York Times,* August 31, 1995, p. A12.

7. Judge Pointer's acknowledgment that the settlement would have to be dissolved was included in the September 7, 1995, message on his settlement information line.

8. Judge Pointer announced the new settlement on his recorded information line on October 2, 1995. Also see B. Meier, "Three Implant Companies Offer New Settlement," *New York Times,* October 3, 1995, p. A14.

9. See B. Meier, "Three Implant Companies Offer New Settlement," *New York Times,* October 3, 1995, p. A14.

10. For a more complete discussion, see Chapter 5.

11. For more on the Hopkins case, see Chapter 6.

12. For more on this topic, see Chapter 1.

13. See Dr. Kessler's August 1, 1995, testimony before the Subcommittee on Human Resources and Intergovernmental Relations of the Committee on Government Reform and Oversight of the U.S. House of Representatives.

14. See comments by Richard Laminack in D. R. Olmos and H. Weinstein, "Breast Implant Settlement in Peril," *Los Angeles Times,* May 5, 1995, p. A1.

15. See K. Rothman et al., "Teratogenicity of High Vitamin A Intake," *New England Journal of Medicine,* 333 (1995):1369–73.

16. See C. Vanchieri, "European Surgeons Call for Independence from U.S. Food and Drug Administration," *Journal of the National Cancer Institute,* 85 (March 3, 1993):353–54.

17. See "Health Ministry Ends Moratorium on Silicone Breast Implants," AP, February 28, 1995. See also French Ministry of Social Affairs press release of January 24, 1995: "Objet: protheses mammaires implantables."

18. The French government announced the reinstated ban in May 1995. See *Journal Officiel de la Republique Française,* May 17, 1995.

19. See J. J. B. Tinkler et al., "Evidence for an Association between the Implantation of Silicones and Connective Tissue Disease" (London: Department of Health, Medical Devices Directorate, February 1993).

20. See D. M. Gott and J. J. B. Tinkler, "Silicone Implants and Connective Tissue Disease" (London: Medical Devices Agency, December 1994).

21. "The Strange World of Implants," *Washington Post,* October 9, 1995, p. A26.

22. See B. Schwartz, *The Costs of Living: How Market Freedom Erodes the Best Things in Life* (New York: W. W. Norton, 1994).

INDEX